T0384986

Toni's warmth, wisdom and years of experience shine through on every page of this book. We humans can find death difficult. The process of dying is often an aversive one in western culture, and therapists working in this space can feel overwhelmed and burnt out. Using Acceptance and Commitment Theray, Toni extends her hand and gently walks us through a way to work with clients facing the end of their life that creates an experience full of value, meaning and vitality. It is an excellent and important addition to the ACT library.

Julie Grove, *psychologist, ACT Therapist*

This book is essential reading for any practitioner who would like to support people at the end of life. Through her wealth of experience, Toni is able to apply the ACT ideas to issues that arise at the end of life and also demonstrate how they are used in clinical practice to help clients live meaningfully. She has a real gift in distilling complex and abstract concepts into everyday language that every client (and therapist) will under-stand. This informative and down-to-earth book will leave every practitioner, no matter the stage of career, left with a plethora of practical strategies on how to support clients (and themselves) when working at the end of life.

Dr. Iris Bartula, *clinical psychologist (psycho-oncology), ACT Practitioner*

Toni Lindsay's experience of working with people facing imminent death is shared eloquently in these pages. The underlying theme of acceptance is balanced with real-life examples of walking alongside someone facing death while looking for what they can teach us about thinking the unthinkable. I highly recommend the wisdom contained within this book to students and practitioners of all disciplines.

Professor Daniel Kelly, *Royal College of Nursing Chair of Nursing Research, Cardiff University*

With deep humanity and humility, Toni Lindsay deftly walks the reader through many facets of using ACT to work with people at the end of life. Dr. Lindsay's impressive ability to bring evidence-based strategies to life through her rich tapestry of clinical experience is a gift for both the therapist and patient and results in a guidebook that can enrich the practice of any psychologist or therapist working with people at the end of life.

Ursula Sansom-Daly, PhD, *director of the Behavioural Sciences Unit, University of New South Wales*

ACT at the End

ACT at the End is based on the principles of Acceptance and Commitment Therapy (ACT), and while it has a grounding in research, it is also a hands-on clinical guide for those working with people at a tricky and complex time of life. This treatment manual is arranged to support clinicians in stepping through common concerns and addressing the ways that people at this stage of life may require psychological support as well as strategies for supporting clinicians working in this space. The guide provides a formulated ACT approach to address each element of the Hexaflex, as well as work around self-compassion and using ACT approaches to support difficult decision making.

This book provides examples that clinicians will be able to apply to their own practices and tools that they can use to troubleshoot clinical concerns. It's a helpful companion to clinicians navigating challenging terrain – much in the way that someone might turn to a colleague for advice, it is open and accessible, while still recognising the ways in which that the work is hard.

Dr. Toni Lindsay is a senior clinical psychologist who holds a professional doctorate in clinical and health psychology and has extensive experience in working with people approaching the end of life, particularly adolescents and young adults.

ACT at the End

Acceptance and Commitment Therapy with People at the End of Life

Toni Lindsay

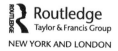

Routledge
Taylor & Francis Group

NEW YORK AND LONDON

Cover image: Thoth Adan © Getty Images.

First published 2024
by Routledge
605 Third Avenue, New York, NY 10158

and by Routledge
4 Park Square, Milton Park, Abingdon, Oxon, OX14 4RN

Routledge is an imprint of the Taylor & Francis Group, an informa business

© 2024 Toni Lindsay

The right of Toni Lindsay to be identified as author of this work has been asserted in accordance with sections 77 and 78 of the Copyright, Designs and Patents Act 1988.

All rights reserved. No part of this book may be reprinted or reproduced or utilised in any form or by any electronic, mechanical, or other means, now known or hereafter invented, including photocopying and recording, or in any information storage or retrieval system, without permission in writing from the publishers.

Trademark notice: Product or corporate names may be trademarks or registered trademarks, and are used only for identification and explanation without intent to infringe.

ISBN: 978-1-032-55617-8 (hbk)
ISBN: 978-1-032-55616-1 (pbk)
ISBN: 978-1-003-43164-0 (ebk)

DOI: 10.4324/9781003431640

Typeset in Palatino
by MPS Limited, Dehradun

I have been honoured to be invited into the ends of
many people's lives – and I have learned more
than could be imagined.

This book is for all of those people, and for those who will come.

Contents

Tables

Acknowledgements

First and foremost, I would like to thank my patients, their families for sharing their stories, experiences and challenges with me – I remain unable to adequately express my gratitude.

Thank you to Anna from Routledge who has taken a risk on this manuscript – fingers crossed that it lands! Your guidance has been invaluable in moving through this process.

Professionally, I have been gifted with working with some incredible clinicians and teams who have shaped both my practice, but also in the ways that we deliver and care for our patients. I would like to expressly thank Catherine Lambert for her ongoing support and guidance. The Psycho-Oncology team at Chris O'Brien Lifehouse – Angela, Katherine, Emma, Sarah, Julie, Haydee, Jane and Gabriella – you all bring such knowledge and skill, it is a pleasure to work with you.

As time passes, there is a core group of people who provide guidance and insight into this world – thankyou to Emma, Fran, Cath, Nicole, Julie, Iris and Sarah. A special mention to Iris Bartula and Julie Grove, who gave feedback, suggestions and guidance to early drafts – the book is much better for your input.

Vivek, Kristyn and Katie, the longer that we work together, the more I see the ways that we care for our patients, but also for each other. To Emily and Karen in bringing together all the bits and pieces that make the AYA service tick.

To the Allied Health Team – thanks for letting me work with you every day, the service keeps shifting and changing, and always for the better.

And for the people outside of all of this – to all of the family and friends – a life is lived in the spaces in between. T, as always.

Preface

My first end-of-life patient was a 15-year-old girl, who I had met in the first days of my oncology role. I knew her disease, and her prognosis, and I had feared the worst as I went to meet with her. But she was nothing as I had imagined, instead she was vibrant with life. We talked and laughed, and we puzzled over how something so small (a tiny little cut) had ended her up in the hospital in such a desperate position. I left the room that day questioning everything that I had imagined about working with people at end of life might look like.

And even though I didn't know her well, I was devastated when she died.

That first conversation was over 15 years ago, and since then, I have met many more people, likely into the thousands who would also approach the period of the end of their lives. Some of the trajectories have been straightforward, but most are bumpy – where the disease doesn't follow the path it should, or that bodies persist against all odds sometimes past the point that their owners want them to.

The privilege of the therapy room, and the space that exists between a therapist and the person at the end of life is so many things, many of which it is hard to put language to – but the thing that is consistent is that the work is complex. Therapy in this space is much more about relationship, and much less about strategy. It is about leaning into hard things and putting language to the unspeakable rather than hiding behind them.

Ever since discovering Acceptance and Commitment Therapy (ACT) it has been the right fit for me in this work. The ways that we show up to our patients is key, and the process of ACT allows not only a framework in which to work with the unfixable, but also in the uncertainty that end-of-life work presents. Furthermore, it gives us a mirror and a lens by which to assess, evaluate and experience our own practice – the iterations of which will move and change as our understanding of the complexity of our own work moves and changes. There is never a point of attainment, instead it is about showing up, even in the face of hard things, and recognising that the space only exists in the moment where it is.

This book is only partially about strategies – we walk through the ways in which specific parts of ACT and the Hexaflex can help to navigate this space – but I hope that in reading it, you take away much more than that. The strategies are the science of what to apply when, but the art is in holding process, connecting with silence and allowing space. Hopefully, from this book, you will be able to access both.

Introduction

Death is the one thing that none of us will escape. And yet, it remains a mysterious beast for many – an unexamined and frequently avoided concept. We have an awareness of mortality from a very young age, but for most of us, thoughts around our own deaths, and the death of those we care about, are avoided. Paradoxically, engaging in reflection and connection with our own mortality allows us to live a richer, values driven life where we show up for what's important for us.

What we can truly know about death is limited, particularly when exploring the concepts around the lived experience of it. There is a strong understanding of the physical processes that surround our bodies as we prepare to die – organs shutting down, breathing changes, predictable chemical and measurable changes that say we are not long for the world. But, it is the stuff around that which is a much more difficult piece. We have no concrete evidence of what happens to us after we die, and as part of our human experience we struggle to conceptualise a world continuing on when we are no longer part of it.

People have been thinking about and writing about these concepts for most of our human history – we have developed rituals and processes around the actuality of death, but the psychological processing of death, and the uncertainty inherent in it, is quite a different concept.

Within the oncology and palliative care space, clinical presentations around death anxiety, uncertainty, fear and helplessness are commonplace. It would be a reasonable assumption that for those who have very advanced disease and a limited life expectancy, they would be the most anxious, and for those with treatable disease, their concerns around dying from their disease would be limited (or at least temporary and fleeting). However, this has not been my experience – the anxiety around death appears universally, and extends further than the patient, causing a ripple effect onto their family and people close to them.

DOI: 10.4324/9781003431640-1

Even outside of working in the acute end-of-life space, many of the clinical presentations that arrive into therapist's rooms will be linked in some way to death – or more specifically the fear and anxiety surrounding death. Uncertainty, or more accurately the intolerance of uncertainty that is commonly seen in clinical populations has strong connections to how we view and think about death, and how we process ideas around mortality.

Whenever I give talks, or present on topics around using ACT at End of Life, people will share their experiences of working in this space – there is often discussion around strategies or tools, but more we speak about process – how is it to be in this space with this other person trying to navigate such a complex emotional experience? What shows up for you as a therapist? What happens for them in managing the unfixableness of the uncertainty that arrives?

This book may appear to have a lofty goal – applying ACT to working with people at the end of life. It will help guide you through working with those who are experiencing anxiety or concerns around death, but is broadly applicable across any domains of uncertainty, anxiety, fear or values based living. It will also incorporate new and challenging ideas around how people may present in this space, how you will approach it and how to amend what you are already doing in ACT to meet the needs of the person in front of you (who may be physically unwell, or doing less well cognitively).

This guide is broken into four main sections:

1. An introduction to the concepts around supporting people in approaching their death.
2. An overview of the ACT model, the Hexaflex and the application of techniques, approaches and strategies when working clinically.
3. An exploration of the challenges that are occur for therapists and clinicans working with people at the end of life.
4. Case studies with examples of the clinical challenges that may occur in this space.

As always, any client discussion is deidentified and changed to make sure that no specific information is revealed. You will see conversations with patients spelled out during the book, these aren't verbatim (my memory is definitely not that good), but instead they are a culmination of many conversations that I have had about particular topics over the years. You will also notice that I swap from using patient, to client and vice versa – the reason for this is simple, in hospital land, people who we see are patients, in other settings they are clients. Use whichever feels more comfortable for you in the space that you work in.

There is also much more focus in this book about the ways that the work impacts on you as the therapist – working with people at the end of life is one of the most privileged positions that you can hold, but the work does not come without a cost. Throughout the book, and in section three, we will focus on how the work impacts on you, how you can recognise the bits that are hard and how the ACT framework applies to that bit too.

My biggest hope for this book isn't that you see it as a manual, but much more as a guide – just as we walk alongside our clients, I hope that this book is able to walk alongside you as you navigate some tricky territory. It doesn't have all the answers, but it is hoped that it will be able to help you find the right direction.

Part 1

Understanding Death and the Psychological Implications

Death will show up in all our lives at one time or another, and clinicians are no exception to this. For many people working in this space, they may find that they have already had considerable exposure to death and death processes, and for others the opposite may be true. Regardless, it is important to recognise that our own experiences with death will look quite different to the experience of working with someone as they approach their own death.

For the purposes of this book, we are going to be speaking primarily about those who have a recognised life-limiting illness and are grappling with the psychological implications of this. For instance, when someone is diagnosed with cancer, or a progressive degenerative disorder. In this group of patients, there are challenging and complex psychological processes which become apparent (such as grief, anxiety, and sense of burden) as they navigate through the process of approaching their own mortality.

Death remains a mystery to most of us – not only the processes by which we die but in the processes around what happens

DOI: 10.4324/9781003431640-2

to us, and our people in our absence. For many people who are approaching the end of their lives, they will be keen to explore these aspects – seeking reassurance and support for how their body/disease/symptoms/medications will impact on them as they move towards their death, but also in wanting to discuss the 'undiscussable'. It has been my experience that many people will only speak about deep fears about their death with their therapists – they don't speak with their families in fear of upsetting them, and often won't discuss with their treating teams in concern that they may be perceived as not coping.

In order to work with patients in this space, it is essential to have a sense of what is expected and appropriate versus what is concerning or symptoms of a more pervasive pattern of distress, anxiety or low mood. The following chapters in Part 1 will step through this – including the symptoms that we see or that patients report (insomnia, anxiety, numbness, etc.), the underlying drivers (intolerance of uncertainty, pain, etc.) and strategies for assessing and understanding process driven factors (such as determining depression from physical suffering).

1

An Evidence-Based Approach

Everything that appears in this book has come from a strong foundation of ACT and using the principles within a palliative care/end-of-life context. Much of this has been borne out of the research arising in ACT, as well as oncology and palliative care for the past 20 years. Throughout the book we will refer to research concepts, works and ideas, as well as those works from other prominent ACT writers (particularly when speaking about particular strategies, techniques or adaptations of ACT principles). To help readability, I have put together a summary of the research in the past couple of years that looks specifically at ACT and end-of-life concerns. It's important to note that there isn't a giant volume of work in this space given the complexity of doing formal research work in this space. Much of what has been developed has come from clinical foundations and experiences, and this book is no exception!

If we explore the general application of ACT there has been volumes of research exploring the use of ACT in various population groups for the management of anxiety (Swain *et al.*, 2013; Twohig & Levin, 2017), depression (Twohig & Levin, 2017; Bai *et al.*, 2020), cancer (González-Fernández & Fernández-Rodríguez, 2019) both in one on one, group and internet-based interventions (Coto-Lesmes *et al.*, 2020; Thompson *et al.*, 2021). The main presenting clinical concerns that are prevalent in the end-of-life population are connected with mood disturbance and the management of anxiety, and as such there is reasonable

DOI: 10.4324/9781003431640-3

evidence to suggest that with appropriate tailoring of interventions there would be efficacy in treating these clinical issues within the end-of-life population.

In the past years, there has been an emergence of exploration of the role of increasing psychological flexibility in the space of palliative care and end-of-life work in order to support patients better in approaching their end-of-life experience (Hulbert-Williams *et al.*, 2021; Martin & Pakenham, 2022).

Several research studies have focused on the role and effectiveness in using ACT with people and their families as they approach the end of their lives. The end-of-life population presents challenges for intervention studies – people are often too unwell for complex therapy when very close to the end of life, or some of the domains of ACT may not be relevant and so in finding global effects of ACT (such as overall impact on cognitive flexibility) may not be reached (Martin and Pakenham, 2022), while other meaningful effects in connection with values, committed action or acceptance may be. It is important to note that many of the intervention studies completed have been on relatively small numbers (which impacts on the generalisability of results) and have focused largely on an oncology population. Several studies have shown that ACT interventions in this space are a well-tolerated therapeutic approach (Mosher *et al.*, 2019; Arch *et al.*, 2020; Davis *et al.*, 2020).

Some of the ACT intervention studies have shown reduction in anxiety (Fulton *et al.*, 2018; Arch *et al.*, 2020) and depression (Arch *et al.*, 2020; Fulton *et al.*, 2018); however, the role of ACT in reduction of pain and fatigue symptoms is less well established (Li *et al.*, 2021). For many of the small studies, there has not been a significant difference shown between the ACT intervention and the control. A recent meta-analysis however showed that across 25 trials the use of ACT in an oncology population reduced psychological distress and showed improvement across the domains of flexibility, hope and quality of life (Zhao *et al.*, 2021) – however, this study was not focused explicitly on those at end of life, where the body of research is smaller. As mentioned above, most ACT studies have been completed in those with a cancer diagnosis and given the similarities across the chronic illness/oncology/end-of-life experiences, it is reasonable to deduce that these same strategies will be helpful. Generally, ACT is able to help people recognise and connect with the reality of their situation, whilst also fostering a connection to acceptance, and value-based living that helps to sustain people through difficult life experiences – particularly those where there is a significant component of physical symptoms. A meta-analysis of psychotherapy in patients at end of life found that across many modes of therapy anxiety is often less responsive than depression, which is congruent with the situation – much of the anxiety is being driven by existential uncertainty (Fulton *et al.*, 2018).

Of the evidence which currently exists, it is reasonable to apply the ACT practices and techniques to the population. As highlighted above, there is significant crossover between end-of-life work and other physical illnesses where the role of ACT has been shown to be effective, and so it is reasonable to extrapolate the work into the end-of-life space. Secondly, the patients and families find that this work is acceptable and is tolerated well, which allows people even when quite unwell to engage. And thirdly (but probably the one with the least evidence) is that it is just a good fit – ACT is all about flexibility, acceptance and showing up for what matters. There is almost no other space in life where these things resonate more than when someone is approaching end of life.

I would encourage you to do further reading and exploration of the research and evidence based on this book (references and other reading materials are listed in the back) to better understand the ways in which ACT principles are applied differently dependent on population, level of physical wellness and exploring domain-based interventions (values, acceptance or cognitive flexibility).

2

The Psychological Components of Dying

Before embarking on a treatment protocol for managing presentations in this space it is first important to understand the common and expected emotions and experiences that are likely to show up for people. Of course, it is difficult to encapsulate all experiences, however, those listed below are the most common.

It is important to note that like most experiences within human psychology, the presentations that you may see will vary widely, and with experience therapists will develop a sense of parameters of coping vs not coping (or problematic vs expected). I have tried to explain as best that I can around this, but often making these distinctions is subtle, and the clinician will ultimately use their skill and experience to understand this better.

It is important to say that there are a range of expected emotions and thoughts that will arise anytime a person is confronted with their own mortality. For the most part, these are feelings around anxiety, uncertainty, hopelessness, loss, grief and general bewilderment. Depending on the context and depending on the person that you are seeing they may have done some work in recognising these as 'normal' and expected, or conversely may be fighting hard to not experience any of the difficult emotions that have shown up. There are significant cultural, internal external influences which will impact how

DOI: 10.4324/9781003431640-4

people identify their coping. It is important to recognise that for many people the default way of trying to make sense of mortality is around avoidance and trying to deny its presence. We will speak more about these folk a little bit further in Chapter 'Thought Management and Defusion', but for now, it is important to be aware that not everyone who presents to therapy at this time may be open to discussion and exploration around the themes of death and dying.

In the first days of finding out about their situation, most people will describe a sense of numbness, disconnection and will often find it difficult to connect with any emotions and thoughts. This can vary somewhat depending on the trajectory to receiving this news – those who have had long illnesses and progressive decline may experience this quite differently to the fit and healthy person who went to see their family doctor for routine tests to find something very sinister.

With clients, I have often found it helpful to name this period of time as the '72 hour window' – being the time that it takes to process and attempt to make sense of. For instance, just this week, I met a young man for the first time only a couple of hours after he was told his cancer had progressed. That wasn't why he was coming to see me, he had been having trouble sleeping in the lead-up to his scans, and had made contact for an appointment that afternoon while he was in the hospital. In between us organising the appointment in the morning and our actual appointment, he had seen his oncologist who gave him the news of a very guarded prognosis.

Our session contained very few words. I watched as he oscillated between hope that he might be able to escape this somehow, to questioning the sense of numbness in his arms and legs that had only arrived after the conversation. As we spoke, he booked tickets to a concert more than 18 months away and joked that he needed to live that long. But mostly, he just looked at the space above my chair and shook his head. How would he ever make sense of this?

But I feel very comfortable that in the weeks and months to come, he will find a way. His brain will help him process the reality, as his body gives subtle signs that things are not what they previously were. He may spend time trying to connect with his reality, but he will likely spend considerable time trying to disconnect from it. He will likely change how he is in the day to day, but these changes will be small ones – it isn't likely to be grand trips or huge gestures. Instead, it will be more conversations with the people he cares about, or sitting in the sun and watching a bird play in the yard.

But more about all that later.

The Threat of a Shortened Life vs the Reality

It wouldn't be an unreasonable expectation that those who have been told they have a very limited life expectancy would be those who struggle the most. And sometimes this is the case. But much more often, it is the people who know that there is a possibility they will be told this information in the future who, in my experience at least, are more distressed. There are several reasons for this – not the least of which is around uncertainty. We are always better able to manage when we are 'in' something vs anticipating being 'in' something. And dying it seems is no exception.

For those in the anticipation phase (i.e., they know that there is a better-than-nothing chance of things getting worse) there is an increased awareness and concern about what is going to happen, how it might occur and trying to plan to manage these things. This may be based in emotions or thoughts, but could equally be concern over practical worries. These practical worries will likely vary widely, but can often be based around pain, money, being a burden, care responsibilities or where they want to die. It isn't uncommon that worries about family, and family relationships will show up at this time.

But knowing that such news might be delivered at some point in the future is enough to make most people anxious. Most will be able to identify the uncertainty about the future as the cause of this, but for others, it may arrive as hypervigilance of medical symptoms, somatic complaints, generalised anxiety or irritability in relationships.

Most people who I have met approaching the end of their lives will recognise that when they have been given the news that they have limited time, they are simply in that space, and they don't have to worry about being in that space. We will talk more about secondary worries and recognising these in Chapter 'Self as Context'.

Don't get me wrong – having the news of limited life expectancy confirmed does not remove distress or anxiety about the situation. But, it does relieve the anxiety and distress about the uncertainty of whether it might happen. For the people who find themselves in these situations, we would absolutely expect emotions and worries to occur, but they will likely look a little different to those explored in the past, or for those who are still sitting in the uncertainty.

There are no correct or standard ways in which people do process this, and it is important that we as therapists show up with openness to this. Anticipating how a session may go, or bringing a sense of how you expect someone to respond in session may in itself impact the direction of the session, and confirm/deny the experience that they are having. Mortality, and conversations around mortality, are very loaded – and probably for most people who walk in the door to see a therapist, they have likely experienced being shut down by the people around them, and it is important that we do not follow the same path.

I Will Give an Example

A patient of mine some time ago now, knew that she was dying. She had done considerable work in deciding which treatments she would accept, and what toxicities felt acceptable to her. We had spoken openly about this, including managing the complexity of what it would mean to 'not do anything' in the face of disease (we will speak more about this in a little while), and she had been able to accept that there would be difficulty in this. She could acknowledge that she didn't want her ability to live the remaining life she had to be compromised by treatments that she felt would be futile. What she did want to focus on though, was having the time to have conversations and say what needed to be said to the people who were important to her. In our sessions we had spoken at length about her belongings and what she would want to do with them – who did she want to give her treasured items to, and how would she communicate with them about it.

The way that she decided to manage this was to meet with each person in a place that meant something to their relationship. And she imagined that she would hand over the object or possession, and they would have a conversation about what they meant to each other, and the role the relationship had played in both of their lives.

Instead, the Very Opposite Happened

For every person she presented the objects to, they shut her down. They wouldn't accept them. Instead of connecting with her in the moment, they said things to her like 'don't be like that, it will all be ok' and 'you just need to be positive'.

Imagine, that we as therapists mirror that process for our clients. We the people who are likely to have some of the most intimate conversations with people around these difficult spaces – and if we even give a hint of the above – a sense of not being able to tolerate the reality, or trying to bring optimism and positivity to a situation that doesn't match where the client is at. Well, very quickly, they will disengage. In this space, more than in others, being able to sit with your own sense of inaction and helplessness is the key (see Chapter 22 for more on this).

What Does This Look Like for People?

Most of the sessions that I have had with clients in this space have had an element of the unexpected. Usually, not in a wild or unruly way, but in the sense that what shows up isn't what I had expected. I have learnt over time that this isn't good or bad, instead, it speaks to the vast spectrum of ways that people process ideas around mortality and their own impending deaths.

The most common ways that people will present are as follows:

1. *Anxiety.* For almost anyone who is approaching end of life, some measure of anxiety will likely arrive (Soleimani *et al.*, 2020). The prevalence of anxiety is thought to increase as people get closer to the end of life, with some studies suggesting that up to 50% of hospice patients experience significant anxiety in the week prior to death (Kozlov *et al.*, 2019). As with other times in our lives, anxiety as people approach the end of life is often strongly related to any sense of uncertainty that people are experiencing. These might be big uncertainties – like where they may die, or how they may die, or it might be about much smaller things – like what time the nurse is coming today, or whether their friends have responded to a text message. There are undoubtedly hallmarks which tend to see an increase in anxiety – such as a change in physical state, increased pain and discomfort or acute transitions at end of life (this acute change very close to the end of life is usually described as terminal agitation. This is predominately a physical experience but will have aspects of psychological anxiety. This is generally managed by medication and palliative care teams, as people are generally too unwell to do psychological work at this time).

2. *Insomnia/Sleeplessness.* Almost paralleling the experience of acute grief, it is common for people to have periods of sleep disturbance and marked rumination at night, with a recent review article suggesting that 50% of palliative patients will experience sleep disturbance (Nzwalo *et al.*, 2020). Many clients can identify the processes around this and can recognize that whilst distraction works well during the day, at night they experience a strong pull to explore the worries and anxieties about what is going to happen to them. Interestingly, clients will sometimes describe this in a very visual way – for instance having intrusive images of them on their deathbed with family

distressed all around them or picturing their own funeral proceedings. Many will describe these thoughts as both simultaneously distressing and somewhat seductive, finding it hard to pull themselves out of them when they occur.

3. *Pain* (or more specifically thoughts about pain). Pain will almost universally show up as part of the end-of-life process (Henson *et al.*, 2020). Most of the time, pain is very well managed by palliative care teams with very specific protocols depending on the types of pain that people are experiencing. That said, for many people, they will have an experience of uncontrolled pain, or difficult symptoms that may bring them into hospital, or in crisis at home (Henson *et al.*, 2020). Expectedly, most people are fearful of pain – particularly if they have had an experience of pain being poorly controlled and unmanageable, which can cause a significant psychological burden (and may impact engagement in activities and processes that help manage psychological aspects to do with the pain). Fear of pain is one of the most common worries reported by people at end of life (Fitchett *et al.*, 2020).

4. *Sense of Burden*. For many people, the physical transitions which occur around approaching end of life mean that they are no longer able to care for themselves in the way that they would previously. This is not age dependent and impacts almost universally. In the process of these transitions, it is very common for people to be cognizant of the impact of their illness on the people around them, and the sense of pressure/weight that having to care for them places on their loved ones. The sense of feeling like a burden is a very well-established risk factor for the management of well-being and psychological health in the end-of-life period (Gudat *et al.*, 2019). Those with a strong sense of feeling a burden are at greater risk of depression, increased suicidal ideation as well as desire for hastened death (Rodríguez-Prat *et al.*, 2019).

5. *Hopelessness.* Approaching the end of life does not necessarily predict the presence of a sense of - hopelessness, however, there are strong correlations in the impact of unmanaged symptoms, psychological suffering and complex interpersonal concerns on the perception of hopelessness. For some the hopelessness is intertwined with a sense of not knowing what the future will hold, and a sense of futility around same, but similarly, it may be that these feelings are tied to particular aspects of their situation, their care or interactions. Unsurprisingly, there have been relationships shown between the sense of quality of life and hopelessness in those approaching end of life – with those with an increased symptom burden likely to experience a higher sense of hopelessness (Salamanca-Balen *et al.*, 2021).

6. *Existential distress.* Existential distress, or the process of trying to understand such fundamental changes to the physical, emotional and spiritual senses, expectedly will arise (Warth *et al.*, 2019). Sometimes, this will be obvious, with clients questioning their experience of meaning, purpose and reconciliation of making sense of a world without them being present. However, for others, these concerns may show up much more obliquely, with anxiety and other psychological symptoms masking the underlying existential distress. It is exceptionally hard to conceptualise what it really means to leave the earth in concrete terms, and for most people, they will struggle with at least some aspect of this.

7. *Joy.* Joy may not be the first thing that would spring to mind given the context, but for many people in this space, an awareness of their mortality, and their limited time means that they are able to see things in the world that make more sense to them than ever. People will consistently talk about the small things that bring them joy, and the simple pleasures that show up in the everyday. They may be able to readily identify what's really important to them, and connect with those things without compromise. For many people at this time, their

lived experience in the world will likely be limited by physical constraints, and it is not uncommon for people to adapt and re-align to new activities and sources of pleasure alongside physical changes. Of course, there are limitations to this, and at times where people are very unwell, there may be very limited capacity to engage in such (Kluger *et al.*, 2021). However, it isn't uncommon that even very close to death, people will laugh with their families, experience genuine pleasure at a cool drink on their lips or enjoy the sound of their favourite music.

8. *Relief*. Another experience which wouldn't traditionally be considered, but is something that many people may discuss. They are of course not relieved by the situation, nothing like it. But, people are often able to identify the ways in which they have been trying to deny the presence of worry, anxiety and struggle about the idea of the 'worst case scenario' (usually this is about death), but then when they are given the news that this is where they are – they are able to see the change in not having to worry about these things anymore. Of course, as I mentioned, it doesn't mean that they welcome the approach to end of life, but it may be some relief about not having to worry about that worst thing anymore.

9. *Numbness*. This is usually short-lived, but it isn't uncommon that people will find that for sometime after they have been told about their situations, or changes in the situation, that they may find themselves feeling quite numb and disconnected. This can be multifactorial – a function of needing time to process such big incomprehensible news, pain or other physical factors and medications which can disconnect from the direct experience (such as pain medications). It would be unusual that this sense of numbness would last for more than a couple of days, but it can take many forms – people may describe a feeling of numbness, but they also may talk about 'zoning out' or spending hours just

staring at the TV. In this space, it can be very hard for people to connect with any emotions.

10. *Disbelief*. Again, this is likely to be short-lived, but can occur commonly for those people who had no sense that things were as bad as they are. This can happen for a couple of reasons – one may be that the person genuinely hasn't felt unwell, and then in some kind of routine way, they find out that they are very unwell. Secondly, it may be the rare person who has no awareness and insight into what has been happening for them (or hasn't allowed themselves to consider the reality of things deteriorating). In my experience, the latter happens very rarely, but the former is not unusual. For those people, it can be very difficult to reconcile the idea of feeling so well, and living their very normal life, while at the same time knowing that they are very unwell and approaching the end of their lives. This will usually shift reasonably quickly as treatment or physical symptoms become more present.

It would be unusual to see someone who wouldn't demonstrate at least one of these emotions/processing experiences. It is likely that they will oscillate through many in any conversation, whilst also moving between thoughts of the past, present and future. There may also be times when complex emotions may show up in combination with others, such as guilt, anger or shame. Like we discussed earlier, it can be hard for people to stay in these difficult spaces for a long time, and so, it may be that they are able to sit and process things for part of the session but will likely move across many domains in each conversation.

As a therapist, this may feel frustrating – and you may be aware of the sense of limited time in a way that the person in front of you may not be. People will vary in when and how they are able to approach or be open to conversations about death, and the ways that these conversations arrive in your clinic room may be quite varied. But, in my experience, it is much better to have many small conversations, then to push too hard to do it all in one session, and then lose the person. It is hard work to do, and thinking of this like a marathon can be a helpful analogy. The people who are in this space are likely to be physically and emotionally depleted, and as such, we need to pace alongside them, even if we feel a sense of urgency.

As we work through the chapters of the book, we will revisit many of these presentations and themes and explore how we may choose to work with them from an ACT perspective.

3

Uncertainty

It would be impossible to discuss death and preparation for death without allowing a considerable space for the role that uncertainty plays. Uncertainty, or more importantly, the intolerance of it, is a key feature in many presentations within a psychological and therapeutic space. Intolerance of uncertainty is a universally recognised experience where people strive to reduce the emotional experiences that arise as a result of an unknown outcome. These events are commonplace in our lives – from interpersonal relationships, workplace situations and health events. Underpinning considerable anxiety that arises from the experience of uncertainty is about one very specific situation – death. As we have been talking about in the previous chapters, death presents us with a myriad of unknowns – from physical to existential uncertainty, it can be terrifying for people to engage in thinking of their own mortality, and most people will actively avoid doing so. Just some of the ways of doing this is to maintain a sense of control, avoid any sense of risk-taking where the outcome is uncertain or become fixated on situations where people feel they are able to be further from death.

So, what happens when that uncertainty becomes a certainty?

For the people that we are discussing in this book, that is exactly what has happened. Through circumstance, they need to explore and examine the biggest uncertainty that we can bump

DOI: 10.4324/9781003431640-5

into. And, for the most part, it is a situation where the tools that have worked in the past are not likely to work now.

There is considerable evidence for the role of using ACT-based approaches in the management of uncertainty – including around the management of death anxiety (see Chapter 1). Any of the approaches that we discuss in Part 2 of the book will be helpful in your approach to working with uncertainty in the end-of-life context.

In a clinical sense, uncertainty (or intolerance of uncertainty) will normally present clinically in the form of anxiety, but will occasionally be expressed in terms of a sense of hopelessness, helplessness and distress around the unknownness of what happens in the process of death.

It is important to mention, although in many ways it goes without saying – that it is entirely reasonable for people to be anxious around the uncertainty that they are facing in the context of end of life. And conversely, the absence of such anxiety would be much more clinically indicative than its presence. For people experiencing it, however, it can be a complex beast to manage, and unlike other sources of anxiety that they have had in the past, it is not something that is easily amenable to strategies.

Many people will seek reassurance and strategies from therapy to try and rid themselves from this anxiety – but at the same time, most will recognise the futility in such an exercise. Likely they have been trying to do everything that they can think of – avoidance, distraction, fighting with the thoughts – and yet it will have persisted. If they can manage during the day, it will arrive with vigour in the evenings, just as they would like to be sleeping. It will wake them and interrupt their thoughts whilst in conversation. And the more frustrated they become with it, the more likely it will be to arrive.

It can sometimes be worth exploring with the client about the nature of the uncertainty. Although the larger existential pieces of approaching death are not problems to be solved, there might be some practical pieces that can be. For instance, often clients will be worried about what happens to their people after they die. Most people can understand that there is an element of this that will always be unknown, but there are likely some things that they can do in this space to help manage this (and to help their people!). Some of these things might be doing legacy work for their children or loved ones, arranging their financial affairs, or making a list of all the passwords to their accounts. Of course, these things don't fix the uncertainty – but it is likely that these things will need to be done anyway, and framing it in terms of ways that they can manage some pieces of it and not others will be helpful.

For the pieces that are too big, or too nebulous to do anything with – this will mostly be the existential stuff, it is really important to name the bigness of it. That may sound strange, but it isn't uncommon that people feel a weight of responsibility of feeling that they need to make peace with or have some understanding that makes their experience feel 'okay' (we will talk much more about this in Chapter 14 on page?). Often people will come into therapy with an expectation that they need to work out 'how to make sense of it' and sometimes there is great comfort in them knowing that there probably isn't a perfect way of being 'ok' with a really inexplicable and unknown thing.

Most people will understand that you as a therapist won't have the answers to these uncertainties.

For some, the knowledge of their 'certain' death will help manage the uncertainty that had been previously present, but just as likely the uncertainty around whether they will die or not, will quickly be replaced by other uncertainties.

Interestingly, in my observations at least, for many people the physical process of dying helps manage the uncertainty, and the anxiety around it quite well. I have observed countless times, the people who have been hanging onto every ounce of control that they could (including micromanaging the teams, and their families) to try and allay the anxiety, slowly and gently allow themselves to be more present to it, and not maintain the fight. Possibly, I suspect, because that fight is exhausting.

But, also, because in those moments it is incredibly evident how futile fighting with something so big is.

Stable Dying

A couple of weeks back, a patient and I had a conversation – six months earlier he had been very unwell, and it was predicted that he would die within weeks. At that time, we spoke a lot about his decision to continue with treatment, and he sensibly made the choice in that moment to say that he wanted to stop treatment and get his symptoms under control. He had been prepared for his death, and so he waited for it to come. And then he kept waiting – his symptoms had improved, but his depression was worsening. He had done the work – the hard stuff around acceptance and saying goodbye, and then he found himself with nothing to do. So, he made the decision to go back on treatment – and within weeks his depression had lifted. In the months since, he had found purpose and meaning again, and the constant presence of death has slipped back slightly from his thoughts. But, he was due a scan – a situation that almost universally prompts anxiety – but particularly for those in his situation where things can change in an instant.

As we talked he was able to acknowledge the strange space of being on a trajectory that was overall heading down towards death – but in the moment feeling quite well, and relieved that his scans had remained reasonably stable.

This is a position that many people find themselves in now – a situation that rarely happened even 10–15 years ago. As treatments change and improve, people are living with life-limiting illnesses for much longer – and having to manage all of the uncertainty that then arrives alongside it. The sequalae of being relatively well whilst knowing that death is arriving soon is a complex emotional space. Although there hasn't been much research in this space as yet, the experience of clinicians indicates that these patients pose significant challenges – complex to manage anxiety, uncertainty of the disease and treatment as well as uncertainty in regards to time, and how to manage hope about the future.

It's hard to know what my stable scans mean – I am still dying, but somehow it has paused, and I am just in limbo

I have conceptualised this idea as 'stable dying' – where the outcome is still certain but in the moment that you are with that person in the room, they are trying to work out how to live. This can be an incredibly helpful framework in which you can navigate values, acceptance and work around psychological flexibility in general.

4

Desire for Hastened Death

Within palliative and end-of-life care, there is a term called 'desire for hastened death' (Parpa *et al.*, 2019). This principle arose early in the development of palliative care, and working with people at the end of life. Desire for hastened death encapsulates the idea of a person wanting a faster death than may naturally occur in the context of an already shortened life expectancy due to medical illnesses of some kind. It is acknowledged that this desire for hastened death may be due to ongoing physical suffering, it can also be a strong indicator of psychological and existential suffering.

The concepts and complexities around end-of-life care and decision-making around this both in the case of the client, and the people who care for them, cannot be underestimated. For most people, the path through this will likely be quite straightforward-they will understand the situation, and actively engage in whatever treatments/medical suggestions are indicated (even if they feel that they are futile) and will be guided by medical practitioners to communicate when they have reached the end of available options. During this time, people may actively engage in other additional treatment options including complimentary and alternative therapies. They may have either actively engaged with, or conversely actively avoided, engaging with palliative or supportive care services.

However, it is important to recognise the complexities and difficulties around managing the approach to end of life. The

DOI: 10.4324/9781003431640-6

path itself is usually not linear – people will experience physical ups and downs, as well as challenges around pain, symptom control and emotional shifts. The way that people cope and manage in this space is also not linear – and as such often ideas around ending their lives earlier will feature.

When I think about most people I meet – I would conservatively estimate that at least 95% of them at some time will consider ending their lives (I suspect this number is probably very close to 100%, but high amounts of shame and stigma continue to exist in discussing this openly). Now of course this doesn't mean that this number of people are actively suicidal or would take steps toward ending their lives, but people will think about it.

There is a very strong correlation between thoughts of ending a life and the experience of poorly controlled pain and suffering – this would be the times when I have had people actively begging me to help them end their lives. However, when that pain is controlled again, or they have time to adjust to changes in their function, this too will generally change.

The rates of suicide in those with a diagnosis of a serious and life-threatening condition is significantly higher than those in the general population (Nafilyan *et al.*, 2023).

The patients that we know are at most risk, are those who are experiencing ongoing suffering. As we talked about previously, the risk factors of untreated depression, hopelessness, and most importantly perceived sense of being a burden are the highest psychological risk factors. In addition, it is important to consider lack of social support as a factor in people being vulnerable to suicide risk.

For many patients, the expression of suicide risk is not about active suicidality, instead more about seeking a solution to a complex and difficult situation. Naming this with people can be quite helpful, as for many people they will be quite scared by the thoughts that they are having, even though they can identify no intention to self harm or end their lives. It can be helpful to frame it like:

I wonder whether these thoughts that you are having are your brain trying to help you. Where you are right now is really difficult, and just like all the other times we have talked about where your brain is problem solving for you, it seems like it is trying to come up with a solution. And so if where you are is really hard, one of the solutions is to not be here anymore. But in having that thought, it looks very different than if you were to actively go out and try to harm yourself.

It can also be helpful to frame as an 'escape fantasy'.

'I don't know about you, but when I have been in difficult spaces my brain does some thinking for me. Like, when we have really difficult days at work, we might fantasise about packing up and moving to Barbados. But that's really just an escape fantasy. I wonder if your brain isn't trying to do the same thing here in making sense of how difficult where you are at the moment is'.

There is also an element of requiring a sense of control, in the face of such existential and physical uncertainty, it makes sense that people would reach for something that allows them to feel a sense of control. It is not uncommon for patients to speak openly about their plans to end their lives if a certain set of circumstances are reached. Often these are physical measures such as not being able to use their legs, or feeling that they have reached a sense of becoming a burden on their families (McFarland et al., 2019).

Many countries now have legislation and provisions for medically assisted dying – this is a comprehensive subject, and not one that can be done justice to in a relatively short space, but it is important to note in the context of how people may approach this. Annecodetley, it appears that many more people undergo the process of engaging with approval to access the medications, compared to those who take the medications. Although the reasons for this are complex and multifactorial, this makes sense in the context of our discussion earlier around maintaining a sense of control in the face of uncertainty.

Risk assessment in itself is something that clinicians are very well accustomed to; however, the experience of sitting with risk in an end-of-life context may feel different and more challenging. These concepts will often raise complex thoughts within treating clinicians about their own ideas of whether someone ending their life prematurely is appropriate or not, and what is the balance of suffering vs choice. The experience of this is also likely to fluctuate and change between patients and can be very dependent on a multitude of factors – the person's circumstances, the person themselves, the therapist's connection to the person and what is happening for them both in therapy and outside (for example recent grief, own experiences of death and dying).

In these situations, it is always advisable to seek support and supervision – as well as doing work on the self to understand the dynamics of the interaction and manage the therapist's emotional pieces. One of the key components of working with death, and especially complex areas such as voluntary assisted dying is in recognising what the clinician brings of their own ideas, experiences and beliefs – but also in thinking about how these intersect with the people that you are working with, and how you approach the complexity of this.

5

A Wolf in Sheep's Clothing ...

Although human psychology is never a simple picture, there are times when the reasons or contributing factors to the way that people are presenting or reporting symptoms can be reasonably straightforward. Unfortunately, this is not the case in working with those approaching end of life. It will be reasonably unlikely that you will be presented with someone for which there is only one problem (or only one contributing factor to a problem), or for which there will be a 'clean' psychological piece to make sense of.

We know that the rates of depression and anxiety in those who are facing serious medical illnesses, including those with limited life expectancy are known to be high. Depending on the studies, this can vary from between 25–50% of all people, with similar estimates for those very close to the end of life (estimates of approximately 40% for both prevalence of symptoms of anxiety and depression in the last weeks of life) (Mitchell *et al.*, 2011; Kozlov *et al.*, 2019). As expected, it has historically been difficult to have a strong understanding of the experience of symptoms very close to the end of life, as patients are rarely well enough to undertake assessments of mood/anxiety. Those of a younger age are more likely to experience higher rates of anxiety and depression symptoms compared with their older counterparts.

DOI: 10.4324/9781003431640-7

When Is It Anxiety/Depression and When Is It Something Else?

It can be difficult to untangle the impact of anxiety/depression in the landscape of complex medical concerns, where symptoms may be intertwined, or even misrepresentative of what the real concerns are. For instance, if I think about a patient I saw on the ward this week – he is a young man with rapidly advancing disease and significant symptom burden. This week medically, he had several complications, not the least of which a wound which has been bleeding consistently resulting in him dropping his haemoglobin (the red cells in the blood that carry oxygen around). When I met with him, he was flat in his affect, reporting a sense of flattened mood, and a sense of hopelessness in managing the situation. Depending on the lens that you apply, would ultimately lead to different conclusions about what might be happening for him.

1. If exploring from a psychological lens, it would be a reasonable formulation to assume the presence of depressive symptoms, and that interventions to help him manage the sense of hopelessness and work around acceptance may be helpful.
2. If exploring from a medical lens, it would be reasonable to assume that the flatness he is experiencing is due to the objective drop in his haemoglobin – the known symptoms of which are cognitive slowing, difficulties managing complex problems and is commonly associated with a subjective experience of feeling flat or depressed.
3. If exploring from a pain lens, it would be reasonable to assume that the impact of the pain of the constantly bleeding wound (as well as the limitations of movement that it has resulted in) in addition to his other numerous sites of pain would lead to reduced capacity to function, and the ongoing nature may lead to a sense of hopelessness in not being able to manage these symptoms.
4. If exploring from an existential lens, it would be reasonable to assume that with increasing symptoms he is becoming

much more aware of the real impacts of the approach towards death, and as a result is finding it difficult to find joy or purpose.

5. If exploring from a medication lens, it would be reasonable to attribute almost all of his symptoms – cognitive, medical and psychological to the high doses of opioids that he is taking to manage his complex pain.

The reality of course is that it is likely to be a combination of all of these things (and possibly more) and so it is dangerous to explore only the psychological aspects of an experience. The example above of the patient's experience is not unique in any way, and so it is worth considering in any formulation to explore the impact of the other things which may be happening around them.

The other factor to consider is that many of the physical symptoms which may occur towards the end of life will have interplay with psychological symptoms. We will talk about pain more specifically in the next chapter, but a good example is breathlessness. Breathlessness occurs very commonly in the medically unwell and is usually multifactorial.

I would like you to do an experiment with me.

Imagine for a second that you can't breathe. Or that you have the knowledge that you can breathe, but it is as if all of sudden your body doesn't remember how to do it.

Most people are terrified by the idea of it. One of the most basic human experiences that we have is that of breathing, so much so that we almost never think of it – that is until something is wrong with it. Because it is so natural and unconscious, even thinking about not breathing can be something that we struggle to do.

So, it stands to reason that when people are having trouble breathing, they will get anxious.

But, if you only try and treat the anxiety, it will likely not be very helpful. As with our example above, breathlessness is a multifactorial problem – there needs to be consideration of both the physical and psychological components to have some improvement in the anxiety around the breathlessness.

What If the Person Can't Tell Me What's Going On?

There is yet another complexity in understanding what is going on for people psychologically at these times – they may find it difficult to find the words, or the language, or the capacity to describe it in a way that we can work with it. Even when people are reasonably well physically, they can identify the challenges of trying to describe the internal experience of facing such existential uncertainty, whilst having emotions and feelings arrive in a way that they have not done before. You may find that when talking with people at this time that the way that they are outwardly presenting looks different to what they are reporting, or they may not be able to answer questions or inquiries about their experience. You may find that many responses are 'I don't know' or some variation of it.

I have noted that a couple of things can be helpful in this space;

1. Give some examples of other people's experiences. Sometimes, giving such an example allows them to identify some of the things that are similar or different for them, and then put language to those things. For example, I might say something like 'some of my patients will talk about feeling quite overwhelmed and disconnected from everything when they get this kind of news ...' or 'Lots of people that I see struggle to make sense of all of this, and so they focus on some of the smaller things around it, I wonder what happens if we narrow this down to just focusing on your sleep for now?'
2. Be silent. Using silence therapeutically is something that most clinicians become very comfortable with, and in end-of-life work it can be particularly important. Often, I will find myself using silence after the 'I don't know' and allowing it to just hang in the air. More often than not, after a couple of moments the person will have found some words to try and describe what is happening for them, and if not, then I will move on. But, for the most part, it seems to help.

3. Allow time and space. Often the work around end of life is a dance of inches rather than miles, and so the thing that the person is struggling with today, may not be relevant tomorrow, or may have a completely different lens applied to it. If you have hit what feels like an impasse in therapy, or the person can't make progress on a particular element, give it some time, and if it resurfaces, revisit it down the track. It may be that at a different time, or in a different context, it may be much easier to work with.

And What If It Isn't Any of This?

There is a reality that for some people that picture will never be unravelled – you may never know what the driver is. This can be a challenging position to work from, but in some ways you don't need to know the answers – in this space, the main therapeutic things that you can do are show up and work with what shows up in the room.

Some sessions will be very targeted on the psychological experiences of dying and processing that – but these will likely be the exceptions. It is more likely that the sessions will be a mix and match of bits and pieces – some about medical things, some about symptoms (I have spent more time talking with people about their bowels than you can imagine!), some will be about families and other people, and some will just be about a tv show that they have been watching.

And all of it is valuable.

The people that you are seeing at this time in their lives have very limited time left, and they aren't going to waste that time on things that aren't important. So, if they are showing up and using the space, it is likely to be helpful for them (and likely to be helpful in ways that you won't be able to see).

6

Pain and Somatic Processes

Given the context, it is not unexpected that pain and other somatic processes will feature heavily in the experience of people approaching the end of life. It is not the intention of this chapter to be a guide to managing these things, but instead about recognising the interplay between pain and other symptoms on the psychological well-being in those approaching end of life.

The process of dying is not an easy one – sometimes there will be a sudden end to life – an accident, a massive stroke, or a catastrophic heart event – but for most people that is not the case. Even for those who are dying of 'old age' are not likely to be doing so in a landscape that is free of discomfort or symptoms. All of us have fantasies about simply slipping away in the night – sleeping restfully and none the wiser of our demise, but when this is not the reality, there can be a struggle to reconcile the experience of pain and symptoms.

Firstly, I will just name that the process of palliative care (might be called supportive care in some places) and symptom management is a key aspect of most of the things that we will discuss in this chapter. In my experience in working with palliative care teams, they do a fantastic role of managing symptoms, even in the really complex patients, and for the really complex diseases. They also manage many of the psychological symptoms – not only through drugs and medication management, but also in their approach to working with people in this space, and the ways in which they can provide comfort and

DOI: 10.4324/9781003431640-8

strategies for the question of 'what next'. They approach things in a calm and collected manner, usually strong with pragmatism. If you are working in this space, building relationships with your palliative care team is a very good place to start. Not only can they help your patients, but they can also help you in managing tricky situations.

The reality is though that not all patients will have palliative care support, and you may be working with someone who has very poorly managed symptoms. It is important to recognise the limitations of any psychological or therapeutic work in this space – for instance, if someone has poorly managed pain you are not going to be able to do any constructive therapeutic work until that pain is better controlled. We can work with patients who have some pain – but any end-of-life pain is likely to be too intense for them to work through.

Anxiety and somatic experiences (particularly pain) play off each other very well – although one does not necessarily cause the other, it is very likely that the two will amplify the experience of the other. For example, in the case of nausea – there is of course a very physical experience of nausea, and will often be caused by physical things (such as tumours, medications, constipation, etc.); however, nausea can often be in anticipation of being unwell (we call this funnily, anticipatory nausea). This nausea can feel every bit as real as the nausea being caused by physical reasons, but often the patient will be able to identify the difference. When someone is highly anxious, both are likely to feel subjectively worse.

Pain

Pain can arise for many reasons at the end of life. It may be functional pain (systems not working the ways that they need to), tumour or disease pain (a process that interrupts normal functioning), incident pain (pain the occurs when people move or do particular activities) or idiopathic (happens because of something that is being done to manage another symptom). In the oncology setting, most of the time pain will come from tumours, and their growth into organs and bones. Usually, to manage end-of-life pain, people will require intense pain management regimes including the use of opioids and other very strong pain relief. While people are relatively well, these will likely be tablets or patches (that get stuck onto people's skin for a set period of time) but as the disease/situation progresses medication will usually be given via intravenous or intramuscular injections. Some patients may be on a continuous infusion of pain medications as well as other medications (such as those to manage anxiety, nausea, etc).

Prior to being unwell, people may have specific ideas about what being in pain means. Most of the time, people will describe pain as sharp, intense pains, or dull aches. They may not identify though, that the sense of discomfort, or not being able to settle, may be similar processes or the early warning system of pain starting – it can be important to work with people to help them identify the ways that pain is showing up and the strategies that they can use to help manage it. I will often make a point of mentioning to people if they are moving around a lot, or seem physically uncomfortable when we are speaking to draw the relationship to pain management, and being curious about what happens after these periods of discomfort, and if it is something that can be managed proactively.

One of the consistent things with end-of-life pain is that it is likely to keep turning up – so supporting patients in being proactive about their management of it will allow them to have a sense of agency over the situation.

The part of pain that we are often more interested in rather than the physical components is how a person responds to it. For those who are already ACT familiar – there has been some great work done by Dahl and Lundgren (2006) on the concepts of acceptance and separating the physical experience of pain and the emotional pain that accompanies it. I won't go into lots of detail about this here other than to say that it is important to help people to recognise the ways that their thoughts are showing up to their pain. I will often have conversations with people about the things that they are able to have some agency over – they can take the medications that they are advised to (see sidenote below), they can notice the thoughts that show up when the pain arrives, and they can observe and make changes to their behaviour that happens when the pain arrives.

Now, of course, as per the point earlier – with people who are experiencing end-of-life pain, it is likely to be very limiting, and so doing things around that may not be realistic, and so it is important to judge and make sense of what this looks like for the person that you are seeing. Sometimes though, people may live in this end-of-life space for an extended period of time, and so waiting for a time to be completely pain-free before engaging in activities that are important to them is not likely to be reasonable. It is with these people that you may be able to do some work with.

For instance, a patient that I saw had metastatic sarcoma (a type of bone and soft tissue cancer) and she knew that she had very limited life expectancy. Her disease was mainly in her bones and connective tissues but had not made its way into her organs. She understood that although her disease would kill her – she was also young, her organs (particularly her heart and lungs) were working well, and it was feasible that she would live for an extended period of time with this incurable disease. The pain that she was experiencing was debilitating – she was often presenting to hospital with an acute pain crisis which would result in long admissions. She had multiple interventions trying to manage the pain, most of which would give her some temporary relief, but she was describing a sense of hopelessness around the limited effectiveness of the 'solutions' as well as significant anxiety both when the pain arrived but also in anticipation of the pain arriving. Even when the pain was feeling more manageable, she was noticing that she was fixated on when the next dose of medications was due, and she was avoiding any activity that she wanted to do in fear of the pain coming back. She could identify a sense of 'having a power over it. If I think about it, then it will come back, but I can't not think about it'. In trying to manage this, she wasn't engaging with her family, her partner, or any of the things that she felt were important to her.

This is the space that we can do some psychological work in – for her, the work we focused on was around acceptance (partially about the inevitability of pain showing up, but also about the emotions/thoughts of the pain arriving) and how she could use the times where she had some pain (as it wasn't likely to ever disappear completely) to do the things that felt important, whilst thinking also about what would help in the times when the pain was much harder to manage (this was mostly about simple behavioural/present focused strategies to try and move the focus off the pain).

Sometimes, in this space, there is benefit in getting to 'know' the person's pain – when does it show up, what is happening around it, are there times of the day when it is more problematic, is it better or worse if they are distracted by stuff that feels important. In getting to know it better, it means that you can work with the person around some collaborative strategies to help them have moments of respite, and most of all, to allow them to use some of the time that they have to do the stuff that is really important to them. Part of the problem-solving process may be about helping them to identify the things that they can do, rather than only emphasising the things that they can't – the process of being in pain (and the anxiety that comes alongside it) is that people may become quite concrete in their thinking, and so supporting them in being flexible can be a very helpful intervention.

Other Somatic Presentations

We spoke briefly about nausea above, but there may be other somatic experiences that people will have that are amplified by psychological processes. Again, it is important to note that it is likely that there will be some physical experience that occurs concurrently with the amplification of symptoms as a result of the psychological experience. Take fatigue for instance. Fatigue is very common in almost all people who are approaching end of life for a myriad of reasons. Almost all people will report it and indicate that it will get in the way of them being able to do the things that are important to them. Most people will also experience a worsening of the symptoms at times when they are feeling more anxious or depressed.

At times it can be challenging to tease out the relationship between these factors – particularly in those who may struggle to articulate their emotional experience of what is happening to them. We know that there is a relationship between those with emotional dysregulation and somatic presentations in the general population, and while this also exists in the end-of-life experience, it is much more commonplace across the board rather than just in those with significant emotional distress. As we mentioned in the previous chapter, it can be difficult for people to articulate their experience of moving through this phase of life, and as such, the emphasis may be placed more on the physical experience as this is much more tangible than the internal experience.

For all the experiences that we have just noted, it is important to recognise that they are often invisible to other people and can only be measured in a subjective way. At the extreme ends of these experiences' others may be able to observe behaviours (writhing in pain, vomiting, hypersomnolence) but generally the experience is only known to the patient. If a patient is having difficulty in communicating the intensity or the nature of these experiences, then it can be important to help them identify the ways that they can describe them to their care team or the people in their world. For instance, saying that they are fatigued is not nearly as helpful as telling the team that they are sleeping for most of the day, and cannot walk to the end of the house without becoming short of breath.

As with our pain example above, assisting patients to recognise the physical components and the psychological components is generally helpful. For instance, with people experiencing significant nausea, I will often talk to them about 'stomach nausea', 'chemo nausea', 'pain med nausea' and 'head nausea' – in separating these out, there is the capacity not only to allow the person to see the relationships between them, and how they are showing up, but also in allowing some space between the physical experience and the thoughts that may be showing up. At times it can be helpful to encourage the patient to name the different things different names (these could be comical names, or anything that they would like), particularly focusing on the cognitive experience of them to allow them to defuse from the experience somewhat.

> I wonder what would happen if we called that 'Head Nausea' something – maybe Fred. We know that Fred is the one who turns up and tells you how terrible everything is. He is the one that tells you there isn't any point leaving the house, you are too nauseous. Or he might tell you how hopeless everything is if you can't get rid of the nausea. I think if you can see him, and recognise him, you can have a bit more of a conversation with him. You could say "Thanks Fred. I see that you are trying to help me, but I am choosing to not engage with you today". How do you think that might be?

Almost all of the physical experiences that we have spoken about above have the capacity to be paralysing if people feel that they are not able to manage them, or that there is no way to escape them. Although the work that we do in therapy about this will not remove the physical experience of them, it may allow the person to have some more space about their lived experience of it, and the way that these symptoms are interplaying with the emotional experience of their illness.

7

Complexity of Caring

It would be remiss to write a book about working with people at the end of life without making reference to those who are in their worlds. The topic of carers is enough to fill its own book, but in the next couple of pages, I will do my best to give a quick summary of some of the main concerns and presentations that you will likely experience in this space.

Being a carer is a job that generally no one willingly signs up for. At the time of diagnosis, the people in the patient's world also get pulled into the space of complex emotions, uncertainty as well as having to juggle the rest of the things that they would have been juggling before. Being a carer is hard work, and they often wear the brunt of the unpleasant stuff that comes when someone is unwell, or in pain, grumpy, or irritable. They will likely also have changes in the way that their relationship looks – they may be providing intimate care like showering or toileting someone, which of course has impacts on the way that the relationship functions and how they are in it.

In many ways the carer's experience is different from the patient's, but most notable is the sense of being a step removed. This can result in carers watching their person being distressed, in pain and suffering without having any sense of being able to do anything to stop or fix their experience. For some relationships in particular this can be particularly challenging – if I think about parent/child relationships the parent will often struggle to not be able to 'fix' things for their child (even when

DOI: 10.4324/9781003431640-9

they can recognise that the thing they aren't able to fix isn't fixable). This can also be the case in relationships where one person has been the manager (practical, physical or emotional) in the relationship, and the roles shift dramatically when someone is unwell.

There is good evidence for the use of self-care strategies to help support carers – particularly when there is a long or consistent need for care over a prolonged period of time. However, in my experience, the process of doing these 'self-care' strategies can be practically very difficult, and if not framed well can add to the sense of burden that the carer is already experiencing (another thing to manage). There are a couple of reasons for this – the one most common ones are usually around the practical aspects of caring for someone – it will likely be difficult for them to be left alone, and as such getting out to get some down time will be challenging. And then there is the emotional piece.

Caring for someone is filled with a huge array of complex and difficult emotions. It is particularly common that guilt will show up, and can be very pervasive both around the carer and their behaviour, as well as how they might be thinking about the future. The nature of the caring experience can be isolating, and the emotional experience even more so.

Carers can be torn between a very difficult present, whilst recognising that whatever is in the future will likely be as difficult if not more so. They may have thoughts arise that they are ashamed of, and feel guilty about and it will likely be hard to communicate to these.

To support carers in a therapeutic sense can be reasonably straightforward – once you can engage them in the service. Most therapeutic strategies that we talk about in this book can be equally applied to carers (with a slightly different framing of course). It is likely that when you get someone in the room with you, they will be relieved to have simple validation of how hard it is, and how they can work to recognise their own struggle (we talk about self compassion in Chapter 18) as well as the ways that they can help manage the complexity of emotions that show up.

Many carers are able to recognise and acknowledge the role of powerlessness in their situations – however, this doesn't necessarily mean that they do not struggle with it. The sense of not being able to 'fix' things can show up clinically in many ways – usually around anxiety and having a strong control agenda. However, at times, this may not be evident in the therapy room, but will arise when patients are on the ward, or in their interactions with the team. This might be more focused on information gathering, reassurance seeking and showing extreme focus on particular aspects of the person's care. This may or may not align with the team's goals, or the things that they perceive to be the most pressing. For instance, it may be that a carer is particularly concerned with a particular medication that the team has changed, whilst failing to connect with the much more serious implications of why the medication needed to be stopped (a deterioration or change in status).

Warning signs that carers may not be coping can be hard to spot – particularly if they are only coming into clinic for short periods of time. It may be that it will be you who notices that they are not coping well – particularly if they are attending sessions to support their unwell person.

It is often at times of crisis that carers will get referred to services. These crises might not be medical crises, in fact, it is likely to be the opposite. We know that when things are going badly, people have a greater capacity to just be in that moment and manage what is straight in front of them. However, when caring for someone who is very unwell, it is more likely that this will occur in the context of the ongoing day to day, where the cumulative cost on the carer becomes harder and harder to manage.

As the nature of medicine and illness is changing, it is often that people are living for a long time with complex and chronic issues which makes it exhausting for carers. It can be helpful to work with both the patient and the carer at these times, as well as engaging the other teams involved in their care to see whether there are practical or other supports that will help manage the needs of the patient, and allow the carer some more time to process their situation and identify what will be helpful to go forward.

8

Delicate Spaces

(Religion, Sexuality, Fertility, Where to Die, Hope)

This whole book could be called Delicate Spaces – the frank discussions about death and dying that we are working through are sensitive and complex topics. But within this space, there are other things which will arise – things such as fertility, sexuality, religion and finances. Although within the counselling room, we are well versed in managing delicate topics when they arise, it can be helpful to think about the ways that you may approach these when they come up. The nature of therapeutic relationships when working with end-of-life patients will often look quite different, and boundaries may be challenged naturally (we talk much more about this in section 3 of the book) – and when coming across such topics, it may be that boundary stuff may arise much more.

I have broken this section down into the most common things that you might bump into, but this is by no means an exhaustive list. Instead, it may be more about drawing your attention to the things that may come up, rather than having a sense of what to do in all situations (if only!). In all of the sections below that are about decision making, it is important to recognise that it is not the therapist's job to help them into a decision, or to guide them towards a certain outcome, instead, it is about providing a space in which to work through the

DOI: 10.4324/9781003431640-10

complexity of it, and sometimes to provide prompts to consider things which they have not previously.

Fertility

Depending on the age of your client issues around fertility may or may not arise. In the population of patients that I work with, these concepts come up frequently, particularly around the end of life. These concerns tend to show up in a couple of different ways:

1. The person wants to have children before they die.
2. The person wants to make a decision about what to do with stored material (sperm, eggs) after they have died.
3. The person wants to delay any treatment until they can either have a child or store the material (depending on the medical situation this might be straightforward or very complex).

All of these situations are likely to have some ethical considerations inherent in them, both for the patient, and their partners/ people, but also the team that is caring for them. In these situations, it can be really important to allow the client to have a space to simply talk out loud through the decision making and help them to explore the reality of what things may look like if they are to go ahead, and if they were to die prior to an outcome (for instance, if they decided to have a child with the partner and the patient died prior to the babies birth). These can be hard and confronting conversations, and can bring up considerable distress as the person considers their life without them in it. Most people will respond well to a gentle exploration of all of the outcomes that they may have to consider, and allowing them space to navigate with direction through this is usually helpful. It is particularly important to recognise that in working with these issues, you may need to be aware of competing agendas, differing beliefs, and strong values for not only the patient, but for the people around them.

Sexuality

Whether or not this is a concern for people is incredibly hard to predict. And as such, it is good practice to check in with all patients around sexuality, intimacy and sexual functioning. It is a reasonable assumption that when people are very unwell they will likely not be focused on having sex as such, but may be very engaged in practices around intimacy and connection. It can be important to explore the ideas of touch and connection (particularly for those whose partner has taken on a caring role) and how their needs are being met in this domain. If you are working with partners, these are also helpful domains to explore to help build some awareness of the dynamic in the relationship and how this may have changed.

Loss of sexual function for some people can be catastrophic – for those who strongly identify with their sexual identities, and their role as a sexual being, even in the midst of being very unwell will likely find it hard to reconcile the loss. It can be important therapeutically to give some context and support around the role of grief, and help them to recognize how the grief around this loss is showing up. It can also be helpful to explore the compounding ways that grief is impacting their lives (if they have lost sexual function it is likely that they will have also experienced many other griefs, particularly in the context of approaching the end of life).

It can be hard to elicit these conversations at times. Firstly, many people feel uncomfortable about talking about sexuality and sexual function, and secondly, they may consider that in the context of what is going on for them, it may not feel important to talk about. All that you can do is to show that you are open to starting a dialogue around it – they may or may not engage in it.

Religion and Spirituality

It can be hard to predict when pieces around religion and spirituality are going to show up for people – and as such, it is important to open the dialogue, even if the patient doesn't need to discuss it at that time.

I have put religion and spirituality together in this section – and of course, I recognise that they are very different things. They can be both co-occurring and mutually exclusive, with people expressing a changing weight on either or both as they move through their situation. I have put them together however because the ways of working with them are quite similar.

Firstly, it is important to recognise that clients will come to you with ideas about how they *should* be presenting and what role their religion/spirituality will play. They may identify that the reality and how they imagined that relationship would look like may be vastly different. Or, conversely, their resolve about their faith and engagement with it has been solidified in the space of approaching the end of their life. For some people, if they experience a mismatch, they will be able to reconcile their experience and arrive from a place of self compassion – but much more likely it will that in recognising the gap, they will struggle to make sense of this and may use therapy to navigate the emotions that arise.

Clients may also make assumptions about the therapist and what their beliefs, and belief systems may be. Although this isn't likely to be a barrier to engagement, it is worth considering the impact of this. For instance, almost all patients will assume that I am not religious based on how I look, but may make a very different assumption about some of my colleagues. Like all of the other tricky topics that we have identified it is important to arrive with openness and flexibility to work and support people in these spaces.

The main ways that these concerns will arise are:

1. A sense of disillusionment with their belief system in the face of such a difficult experience. This may be temporary or ongoing – at the time of finding out about their situation they may distance themselves, but then reconnect with particular aspects of their faith over time.

2. A challenge to the relationship itself. They may question the importance or role that their faith will play in their worlds going forward.
3. Becoming much more connected and engaged. Sometimes, this may be at the exclusion of other things, such as family, relationships and connections with the faith-based strategies to manage their situation overtaking all things.

It is important to understand whether or not the person is troubled by these concerns – it sounds obvious, but it may be that what appears to be unhelpful on the surface (such as being fixated or focused on prayer) may not be seen as a concern for the patient. It can be helpful to do work to support them in recognising how these things are arising, and what impact it might be having on them and their people.

Conversely, sometimes open discussions about their belief systems and what has changed in the relationship can be a helpful prompt to reconnect with the aspects of spirituality and religion that feel helpful for the person. These may be things like social connection or engagement, but may also be in using connection with prayer or spiritual practice to connect to the present moment and to assist in managing complex thoughts.

One of the central concepts explored as part of religion and spiritual practices is the question of what happens to us after we die. It is important not to underestimate the salience and emotional comfort that these frameworks provide, both in having a sense of what to expect, but also in reducing the perceived sense of uncertainty. This is equally true for those who have a strong belief in the idea of an afterlife, a reincarnation or that we simply cease to exist. It can be a powerful tool to explore these belief frameworks in the context of a person's distress about their imagined future and their worries about death and dying. For those who don't have a strong sense of this, or for those who are struggling with their relationship to religion/spirituality it can be helpful to explore the idea of the unknown, and the unknown-ness that death presents, and that that in itself can be a comfort.

Where to Die?

The location of death is usually something that people give little thought to until they are faced with needing to make the decision for themselves or for their loved one. There are three main places to choose from – home, hospital and hospices.

Various reports and studies have highlighted that most of us want to die at home, in our own beds (ideally peacefully in our sleep), but the majority of people die in hospital, hospices and other care facilities. There are many reasons that contribute to this, but one of the main ones is that dying at home is hard. It is hard for the person who is dying – as homes are generally not set up to manage the changing physical needs and abilities of a dying person – whilst also being emotionally complex. Hard for their people (particularly those who live in the house with them) to turn their home into a care facility, whilst also managing the caring needs. They are often also left after a person dies – living in the place, sleeping in the same bed, and managing their own emotions and grief.

The decision to die at home is one that can be fraught with considerable challenges. It is common that the wishes of the patient and their people may not be aligned – in either direction. These things can be very difficult to talk about, particularly if there is a sense that it may be a space of conflict. As mentioned above, the process of caring for someone at the end of life at home is difficult and requires all people involved to be willing and able to engage in the process. If working with patients and families in this space, it can be very helpful to have an open and frank conversation about what the expectations and hesitations may be in trying to manage such a task. There are support services such as home palliative care, etc., but a large amount of the caring responsibility including intimate personal care will likely fall on the carers. Many patients for this reason will indicate a preference to die in a hospital/hospice to not be a burden on their families.

Many people die in hospital. The reasons for this are multi-factorial, but more often than not it is a function of practicality. Someone comes into the hospital unwell and does not make it home again. As people are approaching the end of life, it is not uncommon for frequent hospital admissions for symptom management, or pain crises. Depending on the care facility, they may be well equipped for end-of-life care and be able to manage people in the terminal phases of life. If this is the case, there will generally be active engagement of the palliative care team in decision making and planning.

For those people who have had multiple admissions to hospital, or frequent contact with care teams, there will likely be considerable comfort in staying in a familiar place and being cared for by familiar faces. This can be equally true for patients, but also for their families.

Many of the young patients that I see will opt to die in the hospital. Usually, after diagnosis they will have had multiple inpatient admissions and then as they deteriorate will become frequent visitors. It makes sense that when they approach the end of life they want to be somewhere that feels safe and containing, and will often prefer particular nurses to care for them.

A hospice is a similar concept to a hospital, except that all of the patients have a life-limiting condition and the focus is on symptom management rather than life-prolonging treatment. The hospice environment is generally set up to be much less clinical, and to be a midpoint between home and hospital. Hospices, unlike acute hospitals, tend to be quieter, and less frenetic, and families will often feel quite settled in these spaces.

The benefit of both hospice and hospital is that the majority of personal care, medication management and other care needs are managed by the care teams, allowing the family and carers to just be present to their person.

In a therapeutic context, it is likely that you will encounter discussions around where someone wants to die often. These can be very straightforward conversations that are about checking in with someone to make sure that the decision feels okay, or it could be a much more complex discussion around decision making, family and interpersonal conflict and values clashes. Regardless, the therapeutic space may be the only opportunity that the person will have to speak openly about these concerns without fear or worry of upsetting their people and will generally value open and frank conversation about these difficult concepts.

Some helpful prompt questions might be:

1. When you think about where you might die, what do you imagine?
2. If you think about being at home, what would that be like for you and for your family?
3. How do you want to be cared for, and who do you want to do that caring?

We talk more about this in the case studies.

Hope

Hope is another concept that could fill an entire book! Hope, and more specifically the balance of hope, is something that arises commonly in the end-of-life space (you will see the thread of how this runs through the case studies later in the book). Hope can be about wanting an extended life expectancy, which is most people that you will meet. But hope can also be about being pain-free or experiencing a better quality of life with limited time. The nature of hope will change over time, and as people change in their physical functioning, the sense of what they are hoping for (and what their measure of success is) will also change.

Holding hope in therapy can be very complex.

For instance, this week I saw the mum of a patient. The patient is on the ward in the terminal aspects of end-of-life care, largely unconscious and unable to communicate anymore. Throughout this person's long experience with illness her mum has been unwilling to consider that her daughter may not survive. And so, this week in the face of a shocking and distressing picture of her daughter, she has become increasingly distressed, and has been talking with the nurses on the ward about waiting for her daughter to get well enough to take her home. Many people have become very concerned that she doesn't know what is going on, and that she is in denial.

However, in speaking with her, it was very evident that she knew exactly what was going on – it was just too hard, and too terrible to contemplate. And so, she is holding onto the hope that things will improve, and as things feel like they are slipping away, she grasps more and more strongly onto that. She is only able to 'stare at the sun'[1] for very brief periods, and then she looks away to something much more bearable – the picture of her daughter just as she was, and how she wants her to be again.

Different people will have different ideas about what to do with that – do you challenge her, and reinforce over and over that her daughter is dying? Do you go along with it and possibly feel complicit in some kind of lie? Do you tell everyone who walks in the room to tell her that her daughter is dying?

Therapeutically this is a hard decision to make. Neither is 100% right, and both will result in distress. The choice that you make with this will likely also shift from person to person dependent on the relationship you have and the circumstances they are in.

What did I do?

I listened to both sides – I let her cry and wail about the grief of not hearing her child's voice anymore, and how terrifying it is to see her like that, we spoke about how hard it is to see her in pain, but how difficult it is for her to be sleeping all the time, and I let her talk about how she knows that she will get better if she just has some more time. These conversations happened with fluidity, and she shifted very quickly away from any conversation that left her questioning 'what happens if she doesn't get better'. If you didn't know what was happening it would have looked very strange – a woman oscillating from intense distress and acute grief to a conversation about what is going to happen when they all go on a European holiday next year. She is present to and recognise the inevitability of her daughter's pain – because she is on medication the pain is manageable, without the medication she would be in tremendous agony. She could clearly tell me that it wasn't okay for her daughter to be in pain.

In the end, we talked about holding both things – and that it is okay to hold both. We named the role of hope, and that we all need hope, even in the face of horrible things. We named that some of the hope is also about her not being in pain, and she nodded, with small tears in the corner of her eyes. With another patient I might have had the conversation about the changing nature of hope, and what she thought her daughter's hopes for her time would be, but I knew in the moment that wouldn't be a helpful conversation for her.

You may have people arrive who you perceive to have a completely unrealistic idea of hope and what is possible. From the outside looking in, this woman may have appeared to be in this space, but she wasn't – she knows exactly what is happening, and what will happen. But the hope is helping her to survive in it – and it is never our role to take that away from people.

It is clinically very rare that we will encounter people who are truly in denial – those people are not turning up to hospitals, or engaging in care generally, or if they do, it will be when their disease is so progressed that they are unable to avoid it any further.

In managing hope in a clinical setting, the most important thing to do is to recognise it, and then understand what function it is serving for the person sitting in front of you. It is rarely going to be helpful to challenge these concepts directly, but sometimes conversations around issues can be a helpful thing to do.

For instance, a common thing that arises in those approaching the end of life is engaging in diets with the intention of curing their condition. This happens very frequently in oncology where there are many promises on the internet of specific diets being able to cure terminal cancers. Now, first up, I am sure that if there was evidence for this then it would be widely known and prescribed. Secondly, I am not talking about sensible diet stuff – I will absolutely advocate for that, I am talking about unpleasant, expensive and restrictive diets which have significant psychological impacts on people. There are many and varied versions of this.

Many people undertaking these diets will discuss them in therapy – and the ways that they are difficult to manage. Many of these diets will mean that people spend hours each day preparing food in particular ways, or that they will not be able to socialise because of the ways that the food needs to be eaten or prepared. But, the person will state that there is a hope that the diet may help them when all of the other options are failing. This is a very difficult thing for them to reconcile.

So instead of talking about hope directly and questioning if there is any value to this diet that is hard for them to manage – we might talk about sustainability and what the diet is costing them. We may talk about the ways in which the diet is helpful, but also in what it is taking away from them. And we may also talk about a middle ground – and what would it look like to do the diet for 80%, what turns up with thoughts and emotions and how might they manage them.

Most of the time in this space, the person knows what they want to do, and they need help and support in exploring it. The role that we can hold in that is allowing them to speak through the ideas of what it would be like to shift hope, or to find hope in different things, or to help them work with the values that are underpinning the hope itself (we will talk more about this in the ACT section on values).

Note

1 This is making reference to the idea popularised by Irvin Yalom in his book 'Staring At the Sun' (2008) which explores the concept that thinking about, and being present to one's mortality is like staring at the sun – something that is manageable, but only in brief and intentional ways.

9

Legacy

Or Making Sense of The World Without Us in It!

The idea of leaving a legacy, or the idea of leaving part of us behind even when we are gone is something that most people will have a concept of, as well as need to do the same. The very nature of legacy is varied, and although there may be some common practical things that people may want to do (such as leaving notes or messages for people, recording videos, etc.) there are often much less tangible pieces that will arrive for people in their thoughts about legacy.

For instance, this week I was speaking with a young man about this idea of legacy – he has recently had a recurrence of his cancer and has been struggling quite a lot with the concepts around how he best makes use of the time he has, and how he can make that time important. As we have discussed previously, this can often be a time when people will find themselves getting quite stuck and overwhelmed. For this man, he can identify that he wants to leave a mark of himself on the earth – he wants people to remember him, and he wants to be seen as successful. But as he has realised, and as we have been exploring in therapy, this is a very difficult thing to do, and that is before challenging the notions of how you may begin to measure success in this space.

DOI: 10.4324/9781003431640-11

Legacy is a fickle beast. Even the most famous of people will have a time-limited legacy – if we think about some of the most famous or well-renowned people in our world, most of them will be remembered as people by their people for a period of time, and for everyone else, they will be remembered by something that they have done or said. The people who tend to achieve the sense of infamy are those who tend to do terrible and unspeakable things, rather than those who do good work or commit themselves to a task.

When speaking with this man, he was able to reflect on the death of Queen Elizabeth – a woman who was familiar globally, who had been the standing monarch for seventy years, and was able to elicit a sense of support and admiration from many. But, he also realised that even in the weeks after her funeral, her relevance had started to fade – things move on, there is a new monarch, and people return to the function of their life. And this is how it is for most of us – when we die there will be a group of people who will be significantly affected, and a wider group who will be sad and mourn us, but after a period, people will get on and continue to live their lives – different for the impact we have had on them, but continuing on nonetheless.

Depending on how someone examines this it may be incredibly liberating or conversely, filled with a sense of existential dread and complexity.

The young man I was talking with couldn't see the liberation – and it was the dread that was keeping him up at night. We spoke at length about the ways in which his legacy may not be one of concrete things (successes or accomplishments) but perhaps about those which he has no measure of – the invisible ripples – that are about memories, or a feeling that he has left someone with. These are also things which will be largely unknown which is a challenging concept.

Irvin Yalom has spoken extensively about the concept of rippling – that is the ways in which our lives have influence on others, like throwing a rock in a pond. Some of these impacts can be obvious and clear to us and the people around us, but just as often we are oblivious to these ripples. At times it can be important for us to remind clients of these things, whilst also recognising them in our own work. We, too, have no measure of the impact or lingering effects that our sessions and interventions may have on the people we speak to, and particularly in the end-of-life context examining this for ourselves can be a worthwhile exercise (especially if feeling stuck or unsure of where you are going with someone).

Legacy work is really hard to do. Even for those who can identify that they need to engage in particular activities or processes (such as letter writing) they will likely find it very difficult to actually sit down and do the work. And as such, it will generally sit with them, lingering in the back of their mind (sometimes causing anxiety and worry), that it is something that needs to be done, and they are running out of time to do it, but still, they aren't able to sit down and do it.

Over the years, I have had some patients who would arrive at the first session with an explicit goal of wanting to do this work. They will have clear plans – a letter for their child every year for the next ten years, or birthday cards for all the significant birthdays or recording a series of videos for their partner. They will tell me about how they are going to do it, and they will have intention and motivation. But session after session, they will arrive and say that it hasn't been done. They will likely be beating themselves up for not doing it, and with each week that passes their anxiety will grow. If we sit in session and talk about how they might be able to do it (even at times encouraging them to use the time in session to make a start on them) there will seemingly be nothing in the way – there will be a plan, and timing, and a process. But, they still don't get done.

Because the problem isn't about intention or motivation, or some practicality (like not having the right paper, or not being able to use software). The problem is, that in doing this work, they have to face the idea of a world without them in it – and that is not only emotionally distressing, it is incredibly difficult for us to do.

There is no part of our evolution which has required us to do this – our worlds exist as an extension of ourselves, and even if we know logically and intellectually that this is the case, it is almost impossible for us to plan and understand in any real way about what it looks like without us in it. This is particularly true when we properly try to picture the people that we love and care about continuing on without us.

Part of the utility of legacy is exactly that – we are trying to build an ongoing and long-lasting tangible thing that reminds the world (and most likely the people closest to us) that we are still around, and we are still important.

Of course, we know that this happens anyway. We see it in therapy all the time, when people tell stories of people who have died or no longer present in their lives. We see how behaviours, mannerisms and ways of being in the world are passed down between generations of people, and how most of this happens without anyone being aware of conscious of it. We continue people through stories and memory retelling, and objects take on meaning because they have belonged to the person who has died.

However, when faced with their own deaths, it is hard for people to take solace in such things – in the face of such nebulous uncertainty, it is easier to grasp onto tangible things that can be done.

In working in this space with people it is helpful to:

◆ Recognise and name the difficulty of doing the work.

◆ Give suggestions and tips for how to approach it. The things that tend to be helpful are breaking it into small sections, trying not to do it all at once, thinking about what they want to do or say (so that they aren't faced with a blank piece of paper and have no idea what they would want to write), approaching it as they would any large undertaking – have a plan, be kind to themselves and recognise that it won't be linear progress (some tasks/ things may be much harder than others – for instance, doing a will is generally much easier than making a video for a partner about meeting someone new).

◆ Model and help them to develop self-compassion around this (see more in the self-compassion chapter).

◆ Timing is important – the days when they feel good is the best time to do this, and if they find their energy levels fluctuate through the day, find a good time when they have a reasonable amount of energy and enough capacity. This is a bit of a paradox, as the days when people feel the best are often the times when they are least likely to want to do these hard things.

◆ Decide how much is enough – people will often start with very big and complex goals around this (for instance a letter for each child for each birthday until they are 40). It can be helpful to help them work out what is the minimum that they would want to do and to get those things done first. There is a couple of reasons for this. Firstly, it will help to just get started and have something done, but it also makes sure that something is done in case they deteriorate earlier than expected, etc. (You may not necessarily mention this to people, but it is good to have in mind if things do start to change for them. I have had situations arise where someone has done letters for one child and not for the other, and we have had to work together when they have been quite unwell to get the second letter done).

◆ Recognise that they may not get things done – the reality is that for many people who come to talk about this, and who want to get it done, they don't, mostly because it is too hard and they put off doing it, but often, people will be too unwell, or find that the cost of doing it is too much for them. It is important that they feel supported in this as well.

It is also important to note, that you may be the only person who knows that this legacy work has been done and that it exists. It isn't uncommon for people not to name this with their people as they don't want them to think that they are giving up, etc. I will always ask people if they have spoken with other people about doing this work, and if not, what would they want me to do if something unexpected happens. It hasn't happened often, but there have been situations where I have known that someone has written letters, or had a plan for certain things, and they haven't communicated this to the people in their lives. So, always a question worth asking!

Part 2

Applying Acceptance and Commitment Therapy to End of Life

The use of ACT in palliative care and in health psychology in general has been well established. As we have mentioned earlier in the book, the nature of palliative care and end-of-life work is largely underpinned by psychological concepts such as managing uncertainty, anxiety, grief, existential distress and physical challenges and discomfort. As such, the approaches to suffering and acceptance allow a strong framework by which therapists can approach complex, nebulous and largely 'unfixable' clinical presentations.

In the next section of the book, we are going to step through each of the core components of ACT as well as explore self-compassion and its application in this population. This has been written from a very clinical perspective, as this is what in the past has been helpful not only for me, but for many people that I have spoken to about how to apply these concepts. One of the main anxieties and worries that clinicians have when doing end-of-life work is about what to say, or more importantly not saying the wrong thing. The other anxiety is about sitting with the unfixable, and the distress that comes not only from our

DOI: 10.4324/9781003431640-12

clients but from us as therapists about this. Presenting some concrete case examples will not fix these anxieties, but hopefully may provide some examples for you to draw on and consider as ways to approach the presentations you are seeing or are stuck with.

There are great books that outline the background of ACT and the ways that it has developed. The next section is not a repeat of these – instead it is about applying the ACT lens to end-of-life work. If you feel that you are a little rusty on ACT (or are just learning) you will likely get more out of the next section if you have had a revision of the core concepts and principles so that they are fresh in your mind.

A very important and key component of ACT is finding your own voice. I have tried to make these examples and clinical conversations as generic as I could, but the reality is that after doing this work for a long time, I have a strong clinical voice (as will you!) If you read something that I say as a bit jarring, or too direct (or too Australian!) that's okay – think about how you might approach that in your own voice, and how you may apply it to your clinical group. Much of the of the phrasing that we use in approaching these conversations is very delicate, and as such, whatever you say, and however you say it, needs to feel comfortable for you.

We have spoken a little already about the role of the therapists own stuff in working with end of life and this will often come up when people are seeking particular examples of what to say, or specific wording of a strategy or concept. Sometimes this will be helpful, but often can make people worried about doing something 'wrong' rather than focusing on what is happening in the conversation and in the room.

ACT generally is a therapy that encapsulates the concepts of 'process over outcome' and in the context of end-of-life work, this is particularly important. Many of the situations that will present therapeutically are not going to be about finding a solution (in fact almost none of them will be) instead it will be about working with people to better understand the situation, their thoughts about it, and largely in sitting with difficult things – uncertainty, distress, etc. When working in this space, it can be easy to get caught up in the content and outcome stuff, trying to problem solve, and coming up with strategies and interventions to help 'fix' suffering. It can be very challenging to sit in a space of feeling impotent therapeutically (we talk more about this in the next section – Chapter 10). Many therapists that I talk to find themselves feeling like they are spinning and trying to come up with solutions for people. In this process they can sometimes get so lost in doing the 'right' or 'perfect' intervention that they miss what is right in front of them.

Our clients don't come to us at the end of life with an illusion that we will solve things for them.

And so, one of the best things we can do is to slow down, listen to where someone is, be curious and understand the process that is occurring for them. We know that much of the change that happens in the therapy room is directly related to relationships, and this is heightened significantly in the end-of-life process. Having a good relationship will allow the work that needs to be done to be done, including sometimes the difficult conversations that you may need to lead – however, getting caught up in interventions will usually send the therapy in the opposite direction.

As we work through the hexaflex and the domains of ACT you may find that some pieces will feel natural, and others will feel strange and jarring. This isn't uncommon. Many people can identify how some aspects will fit naturally but cannot see an application for other sections. For some people that you see, you will work your way across the hexaflex multiple times, and for others it will be only one or two pieces that will be appropriate. There are some that are always trickier (self as context anyone?) but allowing yourself to become very well versed in ACT processes will make it much easier to navigate through this. We will talk in the next chapter about ACT formulations, and how these can help this process.

In my experience, it will be unlikely that you will do only one intervention or target one domain with people at end of life. There are a couple of reasons for this. Firstly, the presentations that you will see are likely to be varied and change frequently between sessions, but sometimes in session as the complexity of their experience across multiple fronts of their lives requires different interventions and ways of approaching things. Secondly, the people that you are working with will have limited time, and as such, they will expect engagement about whatever is happening for them and will likely have an expectation for multiple things to be covered quickly (this is true for working with people who are unwell in general – if they have prioritised coming to see you, they will likely have a sense of what they want to have covered).

One of the lovely things about working with people at end of life, is that often the social rules become more relaxed – as they have less time, they get to the point, and they will be very forthcoming about whether something is helpful or not. This is a rare insight in therapy, as people will rarely be entirely honest, and can build a great foundation for doing the work that needs to be done in a meaningful way. The flip side of course is that not only is it intimidating to know that you will likely get some very direct feedback, but that you may be forced to evaluate your approach and goals frequently (and sometimes brutally!).

ACT requires us to be open and flexible, and helps our clients achieve the same. We can model this flexibility in our approach to how we deliver therapy, and how we can support and hold really challenging content while the person is sitting in the room with us.

10

Formulation and Consistency

There can be several challenges in coming up with a full clinical formulation in those who are approaching end of life. If someone is known to you, and you have already been working with them therapeutically, the change in their medical situation may require a change in formulation, but it is likely that you will already know considerable information about how they cope, where the challenges may be, and how they will likely work with the news of their situation. However, if someone is referred to you in the context of their medical deterioration or on news that they have been given a limited prognosis it can be difficult to understand what exactly you need to know about the person in the context of their situation, but also in managing their presentation (which may be one of significant distress and acute grief).

There is usually a sense of immediacy required given the context, and as such, it isn't likely that you will be able to take time outside of the first session to formulate the main concerns/treatment plans. In fact, for many clinicians, the first session with someone approaching end of life will likely be only be partially focused on getting a history and assessment, and mostly on the current presenting concerns and coming up with some strategies and formulation on the spot, with the person leaving their first session already well in the process of therapy. There may be some settings where this isn't the case – potentially in the community if a person had been given the diagnosis

DOI: 10.4324/9781003431640-13

of a life-limiting illness but is relatively well and has a sense of time in which they can work through things as they present. However, in an acute setting – hospital, hospice or other services where referrals may occur as a direct result of deterioration – you may find that you will likely need to bring a flexible approach to what is appropriate in the first session.

The Assessment Session

As we talked about in the previous chapter, people at end of life tend to have little tolerance for things that aren't working for them, and as such, they will engage in therapy and the processes around it if it feels like it is worthwhile, but if they feel that too much time is being 'wasted' and things aren't being addressed in the way that they would like, they will likely disengage.

It can be helpful to make sure that you frame the purpose of the assessment session well – perhaps something along the lines of:

> Thank you for coming to see me today. (Insert name) has referred you to see me. Did they explain how I work, or what I do? (usually, people will shake their heads!). I sit alongside the medical teams and help support people in managing the emotional side of coping with everything that is happening. My plan for today is to get to know what has been happening for you, and how you are going with all of it, and then we can come up with a bit of a plan about what might be helpful. Sometimes I will see people as a one-off, but for many people they find it a helpful space to talk about some of the tricky things that they aren't able to talk with other people about. Does that sound ok for you?

Usually, people will start talking about the physical sides of their illness first – this is usually the part that is very tangible, and likely to be causing significant distress in itself (depending on the situation). It is important to allow people to tell their

stories of how their situation came to be, how they were diagnosed, and what has happened since then. This can serve two
purposes – the first is that the client is given a space to explore
their story and reflect on how things have occurred, the other is
to understand what *they* understand of their illness, and if it is
consistent with what you know to be the case.

There are nice prompt questions that you can use to shift to
move into the emotional and psychological experiences that
they are having. These are often simple, but can be a good
transition point for instance:

'Wow, that sounds like a lot to process. How are you
making sense of all this?'

'How is your headspace with all this news?'

'It sounds like the physical bits have been quite hard for
you of late; how has the emotional side of it been?'

Opening the session with a discussion of the medical components can be an easier way to start – many people are used to
talking about the concrete physical experience of illness with
healthcare workers and is much less intimidating than diving
into the emotional side straight away. On top of that, the
physical component will likely feature in the sessions going
forward. Most sessions will likely start with a recap of how
things have been since you last met, and some of this will be
focused on what has changed medically, how they are tolerating
medications/treatments/procedures, what impact their physical experience is having on their emotions and how well they
are tolerating being in their body when it is not functioning how
they would like.

At the completion of their summary of where they have
been, and how things are going, it can be helpful to ask the
question of what they are hoping to get out of therapy at this
time, and if they haven't already, ask them what are the main
things that they are concerned about.

There is a significant role for normalisation in this setting.
Much of what people will present with will be very expected

in the context of their situations, however, they will have not experienced it before, and as such may be quite anxious about the responses that they are having. It can be incredibly helpful to name this, and to provide psychoeducation and validation about the emotional experiences that they are having. Much of the first session may be providing this kind of feedback to the person, much of which they might not have considered before – I encourage you to not underestimate the effects of this.

In order to complete a formulation whilst the person is sitting in front of you, you will probably do an abridged formulation, rather than the complete ACT formulation (it will likely be helpful to do this after the session). To help us do this, I have compiled the key questions to hold/explore as part of the formulation to guide us in the initial session. I have amended this from the Brief Case Conceptualisation worksheet from 'Getting Unstuck In ACT' (Harris, 2013) (Table 10.1).

TABLE 10.1 Case Conceptualisation Template

What is the main reason for them attending the session? What do they want to get out of seeing a therapist?
What is happening physically for them? (These are things that may get in the way of them doing what is important!) – Pain, symptom control, functional concerns, sleep, cognitive functioning.
What is important to them?

(Cont.)

TABLE 10.1 (Cont.)

How are they spending time now? How much of this is impacted by physical concerns, how much is emotional/distress/psychological?
How do they want to be spending time? What is getting the way?
What are they doing with the hard emotions that are showing up? Avoiding – distraction, keeping busy, actively trying not to think about it. Numbing – zoning out, shutting down, hiding away, using medications/ alcohol to manage psychological distress. Accepting – making room for, being present to, recognising the role of difficult stuff.
What's happening with their thoughts? How are they thinking about their situation? What are they thinking about the future? What do they think that they 'should' be doing at this time? How do they think about their coping? How do they think about how their people are showing up for them?
What things are they actively trying to avoid?

Adapted from page 21 in Harris, R., 2013. *Getting unstuck in act: A clinician's guide to overcoming common obstacles in acceptance and commitment therapy.* New Harbinger Publications.

The idea of this worksheet isn't to do a comprehensive case formulation, but instead it is about providing a framework for which you can begin to think through the components of their presentation, but also in allowing you to make some reasonably quick decisions as you move through the first session to understand what they may need/be seeking in therapy.

For example, I would like to introduce you to Susie. She is going to be a client that we follow through the next section of the book, to allow us to explore all of the ACT components, and formulation is a good place to start!

Susie is 47 years old, and was diagnosed with Colorectal cancer four years ago. She had chemotherapy, radiation and surgery at the time. She has been having regular checks with her surgeon since this time, but last month at her latest check, she was found to have a mass in her abdomen. After more scans, she was found to have disease all through her body, and when she saw her oncologist, she indicated that she could give Susie some further treatment, but her disease was now incurable, and any treatment would be about giving her more time rather than fixing her disease. She reports that she has come to therapy because the doctors told her it would be a good idea, but that she wants some support in supporting her kids through the next 'little while'. In the last couple of weeks she has noticed pain in her abdomen, and in her back where she knows that she has disease, and she is trying to convince herself that it is all in her head, now that she has seen the scans.

Susie was initially very shocked and distressed by the news of the recurrence. She reports that just like the first time, for a couple of days she didn't know what to do or think, but then it all 'hit her'. She reports that she started to panic and spent a day crying constantly. But then, when she started the treatment, she has been able to 'not think about it too much'. She has two teenage kids that she hasn't told about her situation, and has asked her ex-partner not to tell them either. She has a good relationship with her parents, but hasn't told them everything that is going on, just that she has hit a 'bit of a bump in the road' and needs to have some more treatment. She reports that her friends have been great, but she also hasn't told them the extent of her disease. She indicates that it is hard for her to make sense of her situation as she feels 'the best she has for a long time' and has been going to the gym and training to do a 10 K run in the springtime. She reports that during her first cancer she coped quite well, and just 'got on with it'. She laughs often during the session, but reports that she can be a worrier, and sometimes gets a bit caught up in thinking about what might go wrong (not just about the cancer). You notice that she moves around a lot during the time that you are together, and it seems difficult for her to sit still.

She indicates that her sleep has been very poor since she got the news, she is normally a good sleeper, but she has been waking in the night, often feeling quite panicked and anxious and is imagining herself on her death bed. She admits that whenever thoughts come into her head about death during the day, she works hard to make them 'go away' but at night, she finds herself unable to stop the thoughts coming, but also, she is getting 'pulled into the rabbit hole' of thinking about what might happen to her.

Susie works as an accountant in a busy role where she has a lot of responsibility. She has not told her work what is happening with her health, and she is worried about how they might respond if she were to ask for time off. In the past they have been supportive, but financially the business has not been going well. She has some stress around money, as she is the sole support for her children and the household. She reports that she would love to just be able to take the kids and travel, but can't see how that is possible. She talks openly about knowing that she will likely get much sicker than she is now, and currently has almost no symptoms, other than some pain that she is able to 'stay on top of'. She does mention that she has had a couple of 'attacks' of severe pain that she has been very distressed by but has not allowed herself to think about what these might mean.

She knows that she should be making preparations for the future, and thinking about what she needs to do for the kids, but she is finding it too hard to think about. She reports that she has sat down a couple of times to do this 'stuff' but becomes overwhelmed, and instead will end up staring off into space, or looking on her phone. Afterwards, she notices that she is very hard on herself about not doing what she needs to do. She doesn't want to worry the kids about what is happening, but indicates that she is spending quite a lot of time thinking about what she should do

If we think about completing the formulation for Susie with the information that we have, you can see that there is still some considerable gaps, but we can start to think about the ways in which we may be able to work with Susie in an ACT-congruent way (Table 10.2).

TABLE 10.2 Worked Case Conceptualisation Example

What is the main reason for them attending the session? What do they want to get out of seeing a therapist?
Susie can recognise that she would like some support in helping her to support her children as she approaches the end of her life. Referral has been prompted by her treating team (not unusual) but has engaged well in the initial session.
What is happening physically for them? (These are things that may get in the way of them doing what is important!) – Pain, symptom control, functional concerns, sleep, cognitive functioning.
Some pain (likely that Susie is underreporting her pain given the context of avoidance, and how she is presenting in session – moving around a lot, difficult for her to settle). Difficulty sleeping.
What is important to them?
Main concern appears to be about her kids and her people. Mentions that she would like to spend time travelling if possible.

(Cont.)

TABLE 10.2 (Cont.)

How are they spending time now? How much of this is impacted by physical concerns, how much is emotional/distress/psychological?

Appears to be trying to keep things as 'normal' as possible – has continued to work and has not told people what is going on with her medically. Some impact of pain and sleep disturbance. Reports some avoidance in managing her situation. Would like to be doing things other than work!

How do they want to be spending time? What is getting the way?
Spending time with the kids – worries about the future, setting them up well, wanting to keep things as normal as possible.

What are they doing with the hard emotions that are showing up? Avoiding – distraction, keeping busy, actively trying not to think about it. Numbing – zoning out, shutting down, hiding away, using medications/alcohol to manage psychological distress. Accepting – making room for, being present to, recognising the role of difficult stuff.

Using avoidance and distraction during the day – keeping busy at work, not talking about her situation, trying not to think about or recognise the significance of the pain that she is experiencing. At night, getting caught up in thoughts and distress around the future, finding it hard to disconnect from same when they show up.

What's happening with their thoughts? How are they thinking about their situation? What are they thinking about the future? What do they think that they 'should' be doing at this time? How do they think about their coping? How do they think about how their people are showing up for them?

Susie can recognise that she is thinking about this a lot during the night or having times where she is 'beating' herself up about not doing enough. She doesn't comment specifically about her coping, but she appears to recognise that she is avoiding the things that she needs to think about, and when the thoughts arise they don't feel very helpful.

(Cont.)

TABLE 10.2 (Cont.)

What things are they actively trying to avoid?

Thinking about the pain and the impact of the pain (so much so that it is likely impacting on her capacity to do other things). Thinking about the future and communicating with the kids about what might happen to her.

Adapted from: page 21 in Harris, R., 2013. *Getting unstuck in act: A clinician's guide to overcoming common obstacles in acceptance and commitment therapy.* New Harbinger Publications.

From this formulation, it allows us to think about where we might start when working therapeutically with Susie. There are a couple of 'hot' areas that may be a good focus to begin with.

◆ Hard thoughts and emotions showing up at night and causing significant distress.

◆ 'Battle of the should's' around how she is engaging with the kids about her disease, as well as legacy making for them.

◆ How she is spending her time – some apparent disparity between what she is doing (spending her time working and being 'normal') vs what she would like to be doing (spending time with and making memories with the kids).

◆ Pain awareness and pain management.

◆ Acceptance of emotions that show up around the situation during the day (working hard to avoid these currently).

These 'hot' areas are a good opportunity to give Susie an on-the-spot formulation at the end of the first session. Perhaps something like;

Susie as we have been speaking, there have been a couple of things that have jumped out at me that we might be able to work on together. I think that the first one is perhaps doing some work about these tricky and hard thoughts that are turning up at night. I think they are probably also turning up during the day, you are just working really hard to keep them at bay – does that sound right to you? (Wait for affirmation from client). The other thing that I have noticed as you are sitting in front of me, is that, and tell me if I am reading this wrong, this pain is causing you a bit more trouble than you might be letting yourself realise – as I am looking at you, you look quite uncomfortable, and it seems difficult for you to sit in one place for very long. Usually when I see this, it means that pain and discomfort is showing up for people. (It is likely that the client will say something at this time, usually acknowledging that this is likely the case). The other thing that I think we could work together on, is to help you make sense of all of the things that are coming up for you about the time that is in front of you – you have talked today about the ways that you are spending time, and I get the sense that you might be wanting to spend this a little differently.

If there are immediate concerns about pain or other symptoms, it is a good idea to encourage the person to connect with their team to see if there are some strategies that they can employ to manage the physical pain in the first instance.

It may be helpful to give some context to the person about the kind of therapy that you are doing, but using a brief explanation is usually enough. Framing can be really important, and most people will find comfort in knowing that there is a structure/plan about the work that you are going to do together. Perhaps something like:

Many of the people we see have difficult situations, and find that the strategies that have worked before for them aren't working quite so well. It might be things like trying to problem solve, or coming up with ways of trying to get rid of difficult thoughts and feelings. But, in this space, that is almost impossible to do, as it is important that we work to make sense of these difficult spaces. So the way that I usually work with people is much more about trying to manage what shows up, rather than trying to get rid of difficult stuff. It might be that we work together to come up with a bit of a plan about how we make some room for these tricky things, so that even when they are showing up, they aren't taking all of your attention and energy.

11

Six Core Processes

Working with the six core processes to enhance psychological flexibility forms the backbone of almost all ACT interventions (Hayes & Strosahl, 2004), and working with people at end of life is no exception to this.

By way of a brief overview, these components are (the following chapters have a much more comprehensive coverage of each of these).

1. Connection to values-based living.
2. Committed action (doing what matters).
3. Acceptance (NB. We are talking about acceptance of the emotion which arises in the situation, rather than the acceptance of the situation itself).
4. Present focus.
5. Defusion (getting distance from thoughts/emotions/experiences).
6. Self as context (thinking about thinking).

There are some of these which will feel like a logical match for the work that we are talking about. Thinking for instance about the components that we identified in the past chapter and the formulation of Susie's presentation, there is some work that would be suitable in values-based living, committed action, acceptance and defusion. It is relatively easy to imagine that some aspects of values work will be appropriate for almost

DOI: 10.4324/9781003431640-14

everyone in this space (including carers), but for others it might not seem so obvious (for instance Self as Context). The next section of the book is about thinking through these, and looking at ways that they will likely show up for people, and how you can apply/explain these concepts for people.

It is important to keep in mind that many people who come into contact with therapists in this setting might not have had any contact with therapy in the past, and so much of the concepts that you will be working with may be new, or things that they have not considered. I often think about how we as therapists think about thinking, and how this is vastly different from how people outside of this space think about thinking! For many people that you see, they may not even have awareness of the roles that their thoughts may be playing in how they feel, let alone being able to recognize the nuance of how thinking about thinking can shift and move things. It probably won't be helpful to use any of the terms that we talk about here with the people that you are seeing – instead, using metaphors, analogies and examples of how you have observed them in their thinking or in managing their emotions will be much more effective. Similarly, it is more helpful to demonstrate and engage people in techniques and strategies rather than describing them. People who are taking a lot of medications, or those who are unwell, or uncomfortable won't have much capacity for complex explanation (or complex strategies for that matter!) so you might find that the techniques that you might regularly use need some amending to take this into account. Thinking about mindfulness exercises is a good example – instead of a 10-minute exercise, it would be reasonable to start with a simple one-minute exercise, gauge how well the person tolerates it, and go from there. If people are very unwell, the focus will be more on behavioural interventions than cognitive-based ones – this is often the case when people are in hospital, where they can only manage very simple tasks for limited amounts of time. These things will make a big difference though, and so even if it doesn't feel like 'therapy' it can be very worthwhile both for the patients and their families.

Within ACT practice it is accepted that you can start almost anywhere on the Hexaflex, depending on the person's needs and your formulation. This is also true in working with this population, but the order that they are listed above is a pretty common sequencing. Most patients will engage readily with values and committed action work, and there will be acceptance work for almost all people you see. From there though, it can be much more varied, and dependent on the person, and where they are at. From week to week their presentations, and the presenting concerns, will change and so being flexible is the key. As mentioned in the previous chapter, it is unlikely that a full session will be focused on a particular issue – you will likely change from one part of the hexaflex to others several times during a session, and may revisit concepts but in different contexts.

It can be easy to be overwhelmed by trying to cover everything – particularly when it feels like time is both short, and very precious. However, the reality is that you may not be able to do all the things that would be ideal, and the intervention will probably look 'messier' than it might in another patient group. This is okay – dying is messy and complex, and so it makes sense that doing therapy around these things can be too – and so when thinking about using the core components, it can be important to think about the utility of a particular intervention in the moment, rather than getting caught up in the structural components of the therapy per se.

The next chapters will step through examples of using each component in an end-of-life context.

12

Values

I have intentionally started with values as the first stop; there are a few reasons for this (we talked about this briefly in the last chapter). Firstly, most people who are approaching end of life will have already thought about values and what is important to them. Even if they haven't necessarily connected with this, it is likely that when they are first told the news, the things that are important will have come into sharp focus, and so this can be an easy leverage point into a conversation. Secondly, there is some commonality which occurs in making sense of the values work (an example below) where people may find themselves struggling to make sense of the situation, but also in making sense of what is meaningful.

It will rarely be helpful to ask direct questions about values. The use of the terminology about 'values' and 'values-based living' may result in people being overwhelmed, as they may not have thought of things in these terms previously. However, it is likely that they will have thought about the ways that things are important to them, or that they are using activities and things to fill their time.

Prompt questions to enquire about this can often be quite simple, and will arise as part of the normal assessment process. Things that can be a good place to start might be:

♦ You have mentioned family and connecting with people several times during our session today. Are these the things that you are wanting to prioritise at this time?

DOI: 10.4324/9781003431640-15

- What are you wanting to do at the moment? Many people find that when they have been given news like you have that they have some clarity of what is important. Are there particular things that you are being drawn towards?
- How would you know what feels important?
- Is there a sense of what you need to do with this time?
- If I were a fly on the wall, what would I see you doing?

There is significant benefit in understanding how people are spending their time when working therapeutically as it can provide very significant insight into the value or weight they assign to particular things. This is even more the case in the landscape of those who are unwell, as it is likely that they will have to manage the demands of the day with limited energy. You can use this discussion to lead into further discussions about specifics and values. You might ask, how they are spending their time? What activities are they doing? What are they not doing? These kinds of questions can be informative not only in a behavioural understanding capacity, but also when we are thinking about values and recognising not only the things that they are doing that are important, but what are the things that they have identified are important, but that aren't being done. This can be a shortcut to working out how caught up in thoughts someone might be (leading to a paralysis of action).

For instance, when I asked a young man the question of 'What do your days look like at the moment?' He answered me quite bluntly. 'Nothing. There is nothing for me to do, and what is the point of anything?'. When we explored further, it was obvious that any time he was spending out of bed, he was just scrolling on his phone (which allowed him to see his friends doing 'normal' things which reinforced his situation). In discussing it though, he was able to recognise that it was more about being stuck. He wanted to be doing things, but he couldn't work out what those things would be when his subjective sense is that everything feels very meaningless. This then allowed a discussion of how he might be able to do small things that would maybe help give some structure to his day, which would in turn allow him a sense of increased meaning. This example, which is quite common, is a good demonstration of ensuring that we are staying alongside the person – shifting too quickly into the process of purpose building and values work would have lost him. But allowing small steps from a foundation of how he is spending time vs how he wants to spend his time is a step into that discussion.

Throughout your discussions, you may also notice and recognise consistent values showing up – it can be helpful to reflect these back to patients when they are struggling to identify them for themselves. If emotions such as guilt or regret are arising, these can also be helpful starting points to explore the underlying value structure.

Regret Minimisation

Although the idea of regret minimisation has come from the context of business and has applications in the corporate world, it can sometimes have a helpful and appropriate engagement when working with people at the end of life. When exploring this, it can be helpful to set up the concept with the person such as:

> In the space of making sense of values, it can be overwhelming and complex, particularly when there is a sense of time pressure. I wonder if we think about this in the context of regret minimisation it might help? In this space, we don't so much think about all of the things that we can do, which is where the paralysis can come, instead it is about thinking about future you, and not holding regrets. For instance, in three months, what would you regret not doing with this time?

For most people, these will be hard things to think about, but often framing it in this way will provide a sense of clarity. This then allows you to work further with values identification, and all of the pieces which may arise around this work.

When thinking about values it can be reassuring for clients to have some reference points to how others have framed this.

There is usually a significant disconnect between what someone might want to do and what feels important to them, compared to what others will conceptualise about that time for them. For instance, clients will commonly report that they are very happy and content to focus on small and manageable things – for instance, catching up with friends, or connecting with hobbies that they enjoy. Whereas the people in their worlds may be more focused on bigger things – trips or symbolic activities. Most of the time, when people are unwell, they will not have the capacity for big things – but there can be a tension when this happens, as others may be pressuring or trying to organise things for them outside of their wishes (which is very hard to say no to). Clients will often speak about the validation of hearing that others struggle with this, and that it is okay that they are happy to do things which do not form big or lofty things. Many people will carry expectations of needing to have a 'bucket list' or something similar, and may present with anxiety or worry if they *don't* feel that it is important to do these things. In this space, reinforcing what is important, and teasing out the expectations of others (or even self-perception of how they thought they would manage their approach to end of life) can be particularly helpful to explore.

It is important to be cognisant when doing any values work, but particularly in working with those at the end of life, that approaching this work may be confronting for some. In reflecting on their values at end of life, it is very likely that reflections on how they have been present or absent in their values from the past will occur. Depending on the fidelity that they have experienced with their values, this may bring about distressing emotions including shame and guilt. If this is the case, it is important to allow time and space to work with these both in and out of session, with a particular emphasis on the role of self-compassion to both past self, but also in current self as they navigate through the complexity of this. There may also be further work to do in this space in the context of exploring values now – when capacity is lower, and the cognitions that accompany the process of engaging in this work.

Another complication is managing values-based activities when things feel that they have no meaning. This is something that will occur much more often with younger people (who are already developmentally at a stage of questioning the value and meaning of activities, and sometimes existence in itself) or in those who are cognitively more concrete (or even depressed). Sometimes, they may need some assistance to break down the complexity of this.

Therapist: So, what are you feeling you would like to do with this time you have left?

Patient: Well, it's hard because I don't know. And there isn't really any point to any of it.

Therapist: Mmm. What would you have said was important before all of this happened?

Patient: I think I would have said that I would do big things. Like go on big trips or to go and do crazy stuff.

Therapist: (Laughs) I can imagine you doing crazy stuff – what kind of things do you think?

Patient: I have always wanted to drive in a formula one car.

Therapist: That sounds really cool, terrifying, but really cool (both laugh). Why wouldn't you do it now?

Patient: (Pauses) Well there isn't any point, is there? Before I would have wanted to do it so that I could maybe think about learning to drive one one day, or to feel the thrill of it. But, I don't think i would feel the same thrill anymore. And, I won't be learning to drive it, will I?

Therapist: So, if I turned up at your house tomorrow with a formula one car for you to drive, would you do it?

Patient: (Pauses) Yeah, I would.

Therapist: And why?

Patient: Because it would be really fun.

Therapist: (Laughs) So, I wonder whether that might be the point. Maybe it doesn't need to be these huge things with lots of meaning. Maybe the meaning is in the doing, and you having fun in that moment?

Patient: (Pauses) Maybe.

Therapist: I wonder if there might be a bunch of these things that you could be spending your time on that are being thrown out because it doesn't feel like there is enough time for them to be really meaningful. Have you heard the expression about throwing out the baby with the bath water?

Patient: Yeah. It still seems strange to do things that I won't be able to get good at, or that dont really have any point.

Therapist: True. But probably if we really think about it, nothing much that we do really has any point. You know, if you really think about it. But we do things because they might make us feel good, or they connect us with people, or because in that moment it seems important to do them.

Patient: That's true.

Therapist: So what might be some of the things that you could maybe bring into your day that are just there because they feel nice, or that they are something that allows you to connect with other people.

This conversation would then likely allow you to move into a more focused piece of work either around clarifying values, or doing some work on committed activities to work towards those values if you have already established what the person wants to spend their time on.

Now, if we think back to Susie, and the conversations that might show up for her.

Therapist: So, in our first session, we spoke about how it might be helpful to do some work about what you would like to focus your time on, and what is the priority?

Susie: Yeah. I have been thinking about that since we last spoke. I mean the obvious one is to spend time with my kids, but even that is hard at the moment, as whenever I think about them, I just think about how I am going to leave them, and they are going to be all alone without me. (Starts to cry) But, then when I think about everything else it is just too over-whelming. I mean how can you know what to do in the time I have. I thought that I would have decades to do all of the things that I want to do, and now, I just have no idea where to start.

Therapist: I can only imagine. It seems like a bit of a paradox, doesn't it? When you have no idea how much time you have, we think we will always have time to do things, but when we have limited time, it is hard to know what to spend limited time on. I guess it is like money – when you don't have much, it is harder to make decisions about what you spend on?

Susie: Yeah, but when I don't have any money, I know I need to feed the kids and pay the rent! (Laughs)

Therapist: Thats true. Maybe it isn't that different, though?

Susie: What do you mean?

Therapist: Well, when you have limited money, there are some really obvious things that need to be done. And maybe, with limited time it might be the same. I wonder if we could narrow down the huge pool of things to the stuff that feels most important, it might be a good guide rope to help. I wonder what came up for you when you heard about the new diagnosis – for lots of people, they tell me that the world narrows and it becomes really obvious what is the stuff that matters. Did that happen for you?

Susie: (Nods) Yeah, it did. It was a strange feeling, it was like all of a sudden the things that I would normally worry about, like work and money didn't seem that important at all, but I had a really strong drive to be with my kids and my family, and to call my friends.

Therapist: And what has happened since then?

Susie: Well, I guess I have gotten back into a strange type of normal, where I know that I am going to die, but that I still have too worry about putting the food on the table, and keeping things as normal as possible for the kids. I havent forgotten about those other things, but they feel harder to connect with, and even when

	I do, it's hard to know if I am doing the right things.

Therapist: And do you know what that would look like, I mean if you were doing the right things?

Susie: (Laughs) That is a good question. I don't know that I would. I mean, I can't imagine that if I picked up and took the kids to Disneyland or something like that that it would make this feeling go away, but I don't know that anything would.

Therapist: So, perhaps there isn't a 'right' way of doing this. But it sounds like in looking for the perfect way, you might be missing lots of opportunities to be doing what's important.

Susie: Maybe that's true. The kids are a good example I guess. I am spending all of my time thinking about what I need to be doing for them to make sure that they are okay, and that they have good memories... I don't know.

Therapist: You mean that you are missing out on doing those things now, because you are worried about doing it right?

Susie: I think I am.

Therapist: Because it sounds to me, that you know exactly what is important and meaningful for you?

Susie: I think so, I am just finding it hard to connect.

Therapist: So what would an ideal day look like? If you didn't have to worry about work, or pain, or anything else?

Susie: I would start with a slow morning – the kids like to take their time in the morning, but I am always rushing them out the door. And then, there is this place that they love to go. Harry always wants to have waffles, regardless of the time of day. So, he could have the waffles, and then we might go to the beach, just to splash around and catch some waves and bodysurf them into the shore. And then, maybe some fish and chips for dinner near the beach.

Therapist: That sounds like a lovely day. It also sounds like something that you could do now.

Susie:	Yeah, I could. It would be easy enough. It just seems so simple, when I am thinking about dying. Is it enough for the kids?
Therapist:	What do you think the kids would say about that?
Susie:	(Starts crying) I think that they would like it.
Therapist:	And if you asked them what they would want time with you to look like?
Susie:	They would just want me to be with them. They are always getting frustrated when I am working, or on my phone sorting our work stuff.
Therapist:	And it sounds like that day would give them everything that they might want from you. Time, attention, you being present to them, time in the sunshine, and waffles. (Both laugh) You know, I think sometimes this stuff feels like it should be really big, but most of my patients say the opposite. They tell me that they get much more out of the little incidental things that fill the day, rather than the big giant things.
Susie:	That's true of lots of life.
Therapist:	It is, isn't it? What would be the other things? The simple stuff that feels like what you would want to focus on at the moment?
Susie:	I don't know really. I think I am enjoying things that feel connected. Either to people or to times and places. Like I went for a walk on the beach the other day, and it was so lovely just being out of the house and having the wind blowing past my face. A bit the same as when I went to see a movie with a friend a couple of weeks ago. It was so nice.
Therapist:	So maybe there is something to be prioritised in doing those things that feel good in the moment, but I am guessing also left you feeling quite relaxed and content for sometime afterwards?
Susie:	Yup. That's true. And I am thinking that I could do the same with my family and friends. Perhaps I could try and do more where we are connecting over something or just able to be in the moment together.
Therapist:	That sounds like a lovely way of spending time.

Now of course, when we look at case studies, it will always seem very clean! In case studies, clients will always give the right answers and get where you want them to go. Real clients are very unlikely to behave in the same way. But the questions and processes will likely be helpful. The central tenants around values work in those at end of life are focused around:

◆ Spending the remaining time that they have doing/ engaged in the things that feel most meaningful.
◆ Managing the paralysis of inadequate meaning.
◆ Helping to identify the important stuff in the noise of being unwell (and the physical limitations that arise).

Any of the work that is done in this space, with these patients will likely lead to the kinds of conversations that have been outlined above.

Troubleshooting Values

Some people are genuinely unable to identify values and what is important to them. This can happen for many reasons:

◆ They have never thought about it before (or have been in situations where it has been hard or difficult for them to connect with this). In these people, it may be that doing some behavioural/committed action work in the first instance (even if this sounds paradoxical) may be able to give you something to work towards when they can connect with the things that they are finding important.
◆ Their mental state is getting in the way. This can happen for people who are very anxious or those who are depressed. If this is getting in the way, it will likely make more sense to start at another piece of the Hexaflex to address the mood concerns and work to increase flexibility and then revisit values.
◆ They are too unwell. This is sometimes the case, although will likely turn up more often when looking at committed

action than values but remains an important concern. When this happens, it is important to understand what has happened for the person. When very unwell, very limited capacity may mean that values change very quickly, and the distress around whether or not they are working with them is going to be a better indicator than any other. If the person can recognise that they are not engaging in the things that are important, but they are accepting this due to their physical experience, then they may not require further input around it. But if they are distressed as a result, then likely strategies around acceptance and adapting expectations may be a good first step in supporting them. This of course will also depend on whether it is fixed or temporary changes in their physical condition.

13

Committed Action

Working with people at end of life is one of the times where committed action can be relatively straightforward. Most people that you will encounter will recognise that they have limited time, and so they will get on and get stuff done. The caveat to this of course is going to be the physical limitations – most people in this space will have at least some change in their physical capacity which will reduce their ability to complete the tasks and activities that they want to do, even if the motivation to do so is high.

Creative Hopelessness

Being unwell takes a considerable amount of time and energy, and so any work about committed action, and strategies around same will have an element of consideration about managing this. Many people will get caught up in the physical symptoms (particularly pain and fatigue) and will have made decisions about the limitations that will play out as a result.

Most of us come from a framework that when we are experiencing difficult physical things (fatigue, pain, nausea) we will retreat, stay at home and wait for them to pass. However, for most of the people that you see in this space, their physical capacity will likely be deteriorating rather than improving, and it might not be feasible to wait for a time in the future when things have improved, or symptoms have passed. This can be a complex and challenging shift for people at end of life to make as they

---

DOI: 10.4324/9781003431640-16

experience the tension between their physical experience and wanting to live the best way that they can.

It can be powerful to use creative hopelessness in this space – but, will likely need to be very gentle. It can be helpful to use curiosity questions about how they are making sense of the particular symptom/limitation and how it is impacting on what they want to do.

For example:

◆ It sounds like the fatigue is very present. What happens on the days when you do things even when it is around?
◆ I wonder what would happen if, even on those days when the fatigue is around, if you did things differently? If you made a choice to go out anyway? It might not be perfect, or the same as it was, but what might you think would happen?

If in the conversation, it is obvious that the physical symptoms are pervasive and there are no windows when they don't experience difficult things then it can be helpful to frame it in that way. Again, gentleness is the key here – there is a fine line where exploring this can cross into being invalidating (and essentially people having the sense that you are telling them to 'suck it up'!)

It sounds like there is no time at the moment where the fatigue isn't present. And that's hard for lots of reasons, but the one that jumps out at me the most is the one where you tell me that you aren't able to do any of the things that you want to do. This might sound a bit crazy when I say this, but I wonder what would happen if you did those things anyway. You might not be able to do them in the exact same way, but in the landscape that you are in, at least for right now, the fatigue sounds like it is a constant. So, you will be fatigued, regardless of where you are, and so, it strikes me that with that being the case, perhaps it would be worth seeing what happens if you take the fatigue with you to do some of the things that are important.

Of course, the person sitting in front of you is likely to struggle with this as a concept, and they may even say that this is undoable. In this case, it might be helpful to do some creative problem solving, or help them come up with some ways that they can meet their needs.

Most of the time, people will naturally make changes to the ways that they engage with their world to manage the complexity of what is going on for them. They will likely reduce the time that they spend out of the house, or might have people come to them rather than going out to a restaurant. A man I spoke with a couple of weeks ago was telling me that the decline in his physical functioning was the thing that he couldn't get his head around – even though he knew that it would happen, he had imagined that the emotional piece would be what would cause him the most distress. Instead, it was the gradual and pervasive failing of his body, and it's reluctance to do what he wanted and needed.

In working with people to support them in moving towards committed action, it can be helpful to really understand how they are functioning and what is doable, not only what they would like to do.

Sometimes people will get stuck here. The intersection of hope and reality can mean that they might be waiting for a time when things will improve again, so that they are able to do what they want to do. This might have happened before, where pain or other symptoms have been unmanageable and then medications or other interventions have resolved it. And this might be the case again, but it can be helpful to work with people in the frame of 'the landscape of now'. A little like the idea of creative hopelessness above, it can be helpful to work with people about what is showing up in the right here and right now, and how they can work with that. In some cases, I might talk with people about the concept of 'if this is as good as it gets'.

"What If This Is as Good as It Gets?"

I am obviously making reference to the Jack Nicholson movie here, but the question can be a helpful prompt. The purpose of asking such a question is to help get the person thinking about how they can turn up *now* even when it is difficult, rather than waiting for a time when things may be better. Unfortunately, for many people in this space, the time will continue to pass, and instead of improvement they are likely going to experience decline, and as such doing the things that are important (regardless of whether these are simple or complex tasks) will probably have a time imperative. Some people will connect with this readily, and this may be what is getting in the way of them completing tasks. But for many others, they will simply be waiting – for things to improve, and even will sometimes verbalise the idea of waiting to 'get back to normal'. The distinction in mechanism in this example is important – this is not about denial or a lack of awareness of what is going on, instead it is generally about (a) being hopeful and optimistic and (b) recognising that doing anything in the current space is likely to feel really difficult.

And so, using the 'What if this is as good as it gets' question can be helpful. Most clinicians will have a version of this question at their disposal. This is a question to be used sparingly and very gently (just like our example of creative hopelessness above, it can be easy for people to misinterpret the context of this if not used in the right way).

As an example:

Therapist: So what I am hearing is that you are getting stuck here. You don't know what to do, and not much is feeling meaningful, and so, you are getting stuck doing nothing.

Patient: Yup. That's right.

Therapist: So, if this wasn't the case, and things were feeling better, what would you want to be doing?

Patient: I don't know. (Pauses) I would want to do normal things, like going and playing sport, or going to the pub with my mates.

Therapist: And what is getting in the way of those things now?

Patient: I feel like shit. And, even if I didn't, after the surgery my body doesn't work properly. What if I go out, and I vomit, or worse. I don't want that.

Therapist: Is it okay for me to ask you a difficult question?

Patient: Okay.

Therapist: We have talked lots about you knowing that you have limited time. What would it look like if the rest of the time you have looks like this?

Patient: It would be horrible. What's the point?

Therapist: I am not asking the hard question to make you feel bad – what I am trying to understand is, how will it be the right time to do the things that matter? You have talked with me lots about going out with your mates at the pub. But, it seems that the physical stuff is getting in the way.

Patient: Yeah, it does.

Therapist: So, and this is another hard question. What if this is as good as it gets? We don't know what is going to happen in the time that you have left, but it sounds like the physical stuff has gotten worse over time. What would it look like if you are waiting for a time for it to get better, but maybe that time doesn't come?

Patient: You mean as things get worse? Then I wouldn't do any of it. And I would spend the rest of my life in my room.

Therapist: It doesn't sound like that's what you want?

Patient: Of course not. I want to be normal.

Therapist: And what if this is the normal – right here where you are?

Patient: It's a pretty f&^ked normal.

Therapist: (Laughs) Well sure. But normal is wherever we are. And, I think what is happening is that in waiting for things to be better, you are missing out on the now. And I don't want to imagine us having a conversation in a couple of months' time where you say to me 'I can't believe I didn't do those things when I felt well enough to'.

Patient: But I don't feel well now.

Therapist: Of course. But, perhaps, even if it isn't perfect, you might feel better for being able to go out into the world, and to do the things that feel important. I wonder if we might be able to spend some time thinking about the ways that you could start doing some small things to move towards that stuff. I am

	thinking little pieces – like going to the pub with one mate for a half hour – my guess is that even if you feel unwell, you could manage that.
Patient:	Maybe.
Therapist:	What would get in the way?
Patient:	Um. Pain, nausea, not having the energy.
Therapist:	Okay. Anything else?
Patient:	Sometimes the anxiety.
Therapist:	How would the anxiety turn up?
Patient:	About people looking at me, staring at the scars on my neck, seeing how I limp in.
Therapist:	Okay. They are big things to be worried about. What would happen if people did look?
Patient:	I don't know, I don't want it to happen.
Therapist:	Sure, I get that. But I wonder whether thinking through all of these things that might get in the way can be helpful. These are the things that are standing between you and the stuff that is important – so if they are going to stop you doing things, we really need to understand why they are important, and if they are enough to get in the way.

Exploring these concepts can allow people the space to re-cognise the components that are getting in the way of committed action, but also in framing what they want to do with the time that they have left. For some people this can be a very confronting conversation, and so it is important to make sure that you have space in the session, and the person is relatively well to navigate it (like most things we are talking about, it is best to try and do this work when people are relatively out of pain and comfortable. If they are unwell and their mood is flat, it will be much harder to make progress in this space).

Linking Values and Committed Action

If we think back to the case study example for Susie, you can see how quickly the conversations about values will morph into talking about committed actions to work towards those values and vice versa. If we play the previous conversation with Susie in the opposite way it may look more like:

Therapist: So what are your days looking like at the moment?

Susie: I am still trying to work full time, I feel like if I am well then I should be. I am doing school drop offs and then my mum is doing the pickups, and then at night I am pretty fried – I am usually in bed before the kids these days.

Therapist: Is that what you want the days to look like?

Susie: (Laughs) No. If you had of asked what I would be doing at the end of my life, I would have imagined more cocktails and lying on the beach.

Therapist: (Laughs) I think we all have a version of that story! I do wonder, though, what would you like to be doing?

Susie: Really, if I am honest, I have been thinking about that. People keep asking me about what I value or what's important. And I can't come up with an answer, nothing seems to be important enough, but I think I would just want to be with the kids. I cant help thinking that they are missing out in all of this. I am always running around trying to get them here and there, and then I am exhausted and in pain and I don't want them to see that, so I am spending more time in bed and disconnected from them.

Therapist: I wonder if the answer might be in what you just said. It sounds like you are looking for big things, when the answer to the what's important question sounds like it is right in front of you?

Susie: (nods). That's true. They are all I am trying to focus on (becomes teary). But, I am also not wanting them to be without, if I can keep working, it will make it a bit easier for us. There will be a time when I can't, but I am trying to put away as much as possible for them.

Therapist: I get that. And, it also sounds like you aren't ready to give up work yet.

Susie:	(Sobs) No. I feel normal there. I can still do my job.
Therapist:	Then I think that sounds important to hold on to for now. I am wondering though, do you think there is a way to be more connected and engaged with the kids without having to stop work? I am thinking simple things, but things that might make a big difference.
Susie:	I have been trying to think about that as well.
Therapist:	What are the things that the kids really love doing with you?
Susie:	There is this card game that they are obsessed with. They are always at me to play it – but I am so exhausted at the end of the day, I always tell them no. And I feel so guilty (sobs).
Therapist:	I would like you to notice how strong that guilt is that is showing up – I would imagine it is really tough to not get pulled into that. But if we can stay here for a minute I would like to dial in further on the card game. It sounds like this is something that it would be important to prioritize. But, you only have a certain amount of fuel in the tank, right? So, I am thinking that in order to play the game with the kids, there might be something else that has to not be done.
Susie:	That is right – there is a limited amount of fuel in the tank.
Therapist:	It's quite funny how we are as people – we can recognize that we have less fuel, you have so much going on, and so much draining the tank at the moment, but yet, we still expect to be able to do everything that we were doing before. It's kind of the equivalent of going for a long highway drive when you know that you only have a quarter of a tank, and there are no petrol stations anywhere around!
Susie:	So, I need to think about ways to conserve fuel, or to spend less of it.
Therapist:	Exactly, so that you can do the things that really feel important. Like that game with the kids.

Susie: I wonder if I could take up some of those offers for people to bring meals in for me, and instead of cooking we could sit and play the game after dinner. I will have a bit more energy.

Therapist: That sounds like a great idea. And I am guessing that there might be lots of those kinds of things – where you can outsource or just let some things go to free up the time and space to do the stuff that really matters.

You can see that in this conversation, just like in the example in the last chapter, it is easy and quite natural to move between the two concepts. As we work through the remainder of the hexaflex, you will see this time and time again where using one concept will naturally morph into another and back again. You may have situations where you will work only on committed action for a session as this might be a space where people will want to get into the practicalities of what they want to be doing, and how they spend their time, but it is likely that this will form a small part of an integrated conversation in the context of what they need in facing the end of life.

Trouble Shooting in Committed Action

There are times when getting people to engage in strategies around committed action will be challenging. Some of the most common reasons for this are:

◆ They are too unwell (this one will keep coming up!). With these patients, it is important to work realistically with where they are at. Even when people are relatively well, their physical state will impact on their ability to do things. When patients are identifying that it is important to focus on the things that they can 'do' you may need to explore deeply to get a sense of what they are doing/ what their capacity is. For instance, if they tell you that they are currently spending all of their time watching

TV – is that because they are wanting to do that (and are enjoying the process around it, perhaps their partner sits and watches with them), or is it because they can't stand up for more than five minutes due to pain and TV is the only thing that they can do comfortably? It sounds like an obvious distinction, but at times people will skip this step and jump straight to the planning of what someone can aim to do rather than understanding what is achievable. It is also important to note that this will shift and change frequently as they deteriorate or develop different symptoms.

◆ They don't know what to do. It can be difficult for people to ascertain what they want to spend their time on. If exploring and engaging with them around this leaves them stuck, it can sometimes be helpful to look at the option of doing an experiment. The patient and therapist can come up with a small thing to try – perhaps getting out of their room or engaging in an activity that they would like to try. Then, set up the parameters of the experiment, and work through with them how they could try it. Then make sure that when they see you again you follow up – what happened, what was good, what was hard, what would they like to do differently? Often the process of starting this will mean that there will be some momentum gained.

◆ They are too distressed and preoccupied with the future – This may be the case when people have just gotten the news about their situation. In this instance, it will be about getting the person into the here and now (see the section on present focus) and coming up with some basic behavioural things to help them manage through right now. In this space, they likely won't have the capacity to think about values or what they want to spend time on. In my experience, these periods of heightened distress are usually transient, and so may shift considerably between sessions.

14

Acceptance

Acceptance is the concept that carries more misunderstanding than almost any other when talking about death. The ways in which we think about death and the processing of death are laden with emotions and thoughts and heavy with existential uncertainty. But often more than that, the ways that people conceptualise and make sense of their death will be influenced by the sense of how they *should* be conceptualising it. This can be impacted by a myriad of factors – their own experiences, the ways that people around them have made sense of it, and even what they have witnessed through movies, television and media in general. The ways that this plays out can be very obvious, perhaps someone will be able to articulate their own expectations about how they should be behaving or grieving, and at other times this will be more subtle – a sense that perhaps they are missing something or doing the 'work' incorrectly.

I have observed this idea of acceptance showing up in the work around death very commonly. There will often be a strong confluence of the idea of 'accepting death' and 'emotional processing' of death when people are working to reconcile everything and to reach a state of closure prior to the end.

There are a couple of components to the work around acceptance when we are approaching the end of life. These include

♦ *The physical* – There are clear and significant physical markers and changes which are consistent with the body

DOI: 10.4324/9781003431640-17

beginning to shut down, and ceasing to function. Depending on the situation, these changes may happen rapidly or in a gradual function. People will often describe a sense of 'needing to accept' these changes, even in the face of very challenging situations. Interestingly, often the real work of acceptance in this space is driven by the physiological processes of dying rather than the emotional process of acceptance work.

◆ *The emotional* – Expectedly, almost everyone who is approaching the end of life will experience emotional changes and experiences. This is the dominant area that we will focus on as we discuss and make sense of acceptance from an ACT perspective.

◆ *The existential* – Similarly to the emotional work above, most people will have some experience of existential processing as they approach the end of life. Although one of the goals for people in doing this work is to determine a sense of certainty, the uncertainty will remain. As with emotional work, the role in acceptance in this space is much more about managing the role of the uncertainty and existential distress than working with acceptance of an outcome.

It is important to be clear with the people you are working with about the distinctions about acceptance. When you speak about acceptance, it is likely that your patient will assume you want them to accept the situation. This is not the goal – we are talking about accepting the emotions/thoughts/feelings/experiences that arise as a *result* of the experience. This can be very complex for people to get their heads around (particularly when they are getting mixed messages from the people in their worlds about having to 'accept things' or to be 'positive and optimistic'.

By way of an example:

Therapist: So, these thoughts that are turning up all the time. How are they different?

Patient: I don't know exactly. They are still the same in lots of ways, they are about leaving the kids and being sad.

I just keep thinking that I need to find a way to be okay with all of this, you know, to accept it, and move on in some way.

Therapist: Move on? In what way do you mean?

Patient: I don't know. It just seems, though, that I can't move past this. If I could work out a way to accept it, then perhaps it would feel more manageable somehow.

Therapist: Accepting what?

Patient: The whole thing.

Therapist: The death stuff? (Pause while patient nods head) How would you know that you have accepted it?

Patient: Um, I don't know really. Maybe I would feel okay about it.

Therapist: You would feel okay about dying?

Patient: Maybe. (Pauses for a couple of minutes) It's just really hard. I can't work out how to do it.

Therapist: (Pauses) I wonder if you might not be able to?

Patient: What do you mean?

Therapist: Well, it sounds like what you are describing is that you want to be 'okay' with all of this. You want it to be okay to be dying, and that you wouldn't have any emotions about that, or that you had somehow worked out a way to process those emotions. Am I reading that right?

Patient: Yeah, but when you say it like that it sounds a bit unrealistic.

Therapist: Hmm. That's what I mean when I say that I am not sure that it is possible. I think for you to be able to do as you are describing, it would mean you not feeling anything about it at all anymore.

Patient: Yeah. That's true.

Therapist: And I just can't imagine a time where you will say to me – 'You know what. I am completely okay with everything that is happening here'.

Patient: (Laughs) Yeah, I guess not.

Therapist: I think what we can do work on though is all of the things that turn up around the thing itself. The

	sadness, the grief, the anger and the frustration. I think that we can do some work around accepting them, and making space for those things to come and go.
Patient:	Let me guess, we cant get rid of those either … (laughs).
Therapist:	Not unless you know something that I don't. (Laughs) I think that those things turning up are part of what makes you very human and speaks to the weight of everything that is going on. Imagine the reverse. Imagine if you were sitting here and saying to me 'I don't care about this. I don't feel anything'
Patient:	That wouldn't feel right.
Therapist:	No. And so, I think the acceptance is about knowing that the difficult things are going to show up. Not about being 'okay' with why they are showing up.

For many people, this will be a conversation that will need to be revisited over and over in various ways. In my observations, people can find it harder to generalise the ideas of acceptance across multiple domains at end of life, in ways that they may not in other clinical areas. I suspect that this is due to the synchronous and rapid changes that happen across their emotional, physical, social and existential functioning, and as such, despite things being very similar in terms of the role that acceptance plays, it may be hard for them to recognise these spaces.

The role of naming both emotions and acceptance is a key component of doing acceptance work. In using naming, such as in the above example, it allows a conversation to be had about the function of the emotions and experiences as well as the lived experience of them showing up. In being consistent about the role of this, it further allows an ongoing therapeutic conversation to take place exploring the different ways that acceptance may be helpful, and in recognising when difficult things have arisen. For example, with our person above it may be helpful to have a conversation such as:

Therapist: So, I wonder what happens if we were to name these emotions – the ones that show up around this. I don't mind what you call it, but I wonder if we named them and get to know them a little better, that when they arise in the future, you can recognise them easier.

Patient: That makes sense.

Therapist: My guess is that they are probably going to hang around a bit, these tricky emotions. They might sit there on your shoulder and turn up at particular times. I think sometimes knowing that they are going to show up means that you can make a bit more room for them.

What Would It Take to Make a Friend?

For many people, the idea of making room and allowing difficult thoughts and emotions to be present is going to be very challenging. It can be helpful at these times to explain (very generally) the foundations of ACT and the work around suffering as part of our natural and expected part of our human experience, but pointing out that the stories that we tell ourselves are often the opposite to this – any sense of discomfort or hardness (emotionally or cognitively) means that there is something inherently wrong. In working with people at end of life, people will likely have more tolerance for difficult emotional experiences, but will likely continue to struggle with some aspects of this. Mostly, these are around really complex emotions like grief, guilt or shame.

A concept to help support patients in making sense of the relationships with difficult emotions, I have found posing the following question to people quite helpful.

What would it take to make a friend of this guilt/shame/grief/sadness (whichever is appropriate) rather than an enemy?

Sometimes, people might be initially put off by such a question whereas for others, they will get it right away.

A further explanation might be along the lines of:

> You know, I always think about the energy it takes to keep something/someone an enemy. There are all of the rules about it. We have to make constant decisions about how we engage with it, and what we do to avoid it. It takes a huge amount of cognitive load and big brain space. And at the moment, you are telling me, you don't have a huge amount of space with the physical energy everything is taking.
>
> When I think of the experience of having an enemy – sometimes, the enemy doesn't even know that they are our enemy. They are just walking around doing what they do – and most of the time they aren't even aware of us. But, on top of that because we are so focused on them being our enemy, we are blind to the other pieces of them, and some of those pieces might be great! It sounds like the same thing is happening with this idea of (insert emotion). It is just doing its thing. And you are carrying all the weight. So, I wonder, just like that school-yard bully, if you could make friends with them, or at least stop being the enemy, how much more space would you have?

The Drunk Guy at the Cricket Match

One of my favourite analogies for acceptance came in part from a conversation that I had with one of my young patients one day (and incidentally, was also one of my favourite patients). He had been a mad keen cricket player, and we were talking about difficult emotions showing up.

Therapist: So, when you are on the pitch, my guess is there is always that guy. You know the one who is yelling unhelpful comments.

Patient: Yeah, there is. Always a bloke.

Therapist: What do you do with him? Do you talk back to him? Do you change what you do because of what he says?

Patient: Nah. No point. He is just a drunk idiot. He is always going to be yelling something at me. So, I just get on and play.

Therapist: Seems to me that that guy is a little bit like those emotions that are showing up. They are turning up when you don't want them, but you can't do anything to stop them either, and so, you end up just getting on and doing what you need to do.

Now, of course, this is a very Australian analogy, and a bit absurd. But I have found that my patients really enjoy it, and it also means that you can have a little bit of fun with it. It goes without saying that the emotions that are showing up around end of life are going to be big emotions, but you can handle this with sensitivity and kindness, whilst still using the same concept.

The Cast of Characters

It may have arisen as a function of working primarily with younger people, but somewhere along the line it has become helpful in the work that I do around end of life to help people to get to know the characters that live in their brains. This isn't a new concept, and I did not by any stretch come up with it, but it is something that most people are able to understand and make sense of.

This can be a really helpful way of discussing and making room for emotions, particularly the unpleasant and hard ones which are showing up. This strategy can work really well for difficult things like grief, but also shame and guilt which can be harder for people to conceptualise. I have started the conversation about these characters here in the section on acceptance, but we will also revisit this concept when we look at defusion and thought management as they go well together.

When you have introduced the idea of these characters into the dialogue, it can be easier to leverage and make other links for people as they progress therapeutically.

An Acceptance Dialogue

Let's revisit Susie – one of the challenges that she was having was managing the emotions that would arise, and her work of fighting against them – a strategy that was working well during the day, but at night was becoming much more problematic.

Therapist: So, tell me more about those thoughts that have been showing up at night.

Susie: They are thoughts about the future mostly, me leaving the kids, what it will be like to die. (sobs). I just keep thinking about how they will be without their mum, and how unfair it is that that is happening to them.

Therapist: That sounds very distressing. (Pauses) Are they the same thoughts every time?

Susie: Mostly. They aren't too bad during the day, but the second I put my head down on the pillow to sleep they arrive.

Therapist: I would like to understand these thoughts better. Would that be okay? It would be interesting to notice how they are showing up. Are they words, or pictures, or do you hear the thoughts coming?

Susie: Um, I haven't really thought about it like that. I guess that I mostly hear them, and then sometimes there are images that come along with them – usually the kids being really distressed, or I imagine what they will look like when they are older.

Therapist: And how do these thoughts stop? Do they have a natural end point?

Susie: (Pauses) You are probably going to think this is a bit crazy, but I have this image of myself on my deathbed with all my family around me. (Sobs)

Therapist: That doesn't sound crazy at all. Would it surprise you if I said that people having that image, particularly at night is really common?

Susie: It would. It's such a cruel thing to happen – there is something about that image that makes it feel more real somehow.

Therapist: Something that immerses you into that space? (Pauses) Why do you think these things are showing up at night?

Susie: I don't know. I think that it is the time when it is quiet and dark, and perhaps I have more time to think about it then.

Therapist: You are probably right. I also wonder whether it might be the time when you are working less hard to keep it away.

Susie: What do you mean?

Therapist: Well, when you have spoken to me about how you are spending the days it feels like they are pretty full – and I am sure that they would be anyway, but I wonder whether part of that busyness is to not be thinking about everything that is going on?

Susie: Maybe.

Therapist: It sounds like these thoughts are really painful, and when they are showing up during the day, you are working hard for them not to be there. But, it seems like something different happens at night.

Susie: It feels harder to control them at night. My pain is usually worse when I lie down, and so I sometimes feel like I just give into it, and it washes over me. (Sobs)

Therapist: (Pauses) That sounds like both ways are hard – the days sound exhausting with you doing everything that you can not to be thinking about it, but then at night when the thoughts come they feel completely overwhelming and out of control. Is that how it feels for you?

Susie: Yeah, it does. I just want them to be gone.

Therapist: Do you think that's possible? To never think about these things again?

Susie: No. What kind of a mother would I be if I wasn't sad or worried about my kids.

Therapist: I think you are right. It sounds like these thoughts are showing up as a direct relationship to the situation that you are in. If they weren't turning up, I think we would both be more worried.

Susie: Mmm. So, you are saying that they won't go away.

Therapist: I don't think so. Almost everyone I meet has these difficult thoughts and emotions show up. And, I don't think I have ever met anyone who can make them go away. I wonder whether we need to shift the focus here. Maybe instead of working hard and being exhausted by trying to get rid of them, we work on some strategies to help make room for them.

Susie: I don't want to make room for them. Then they will take over.

Therapist: It's interesting how our brains go there isn't it? Is that what happens now – for instance at night when you give them space?

Susie: Kind of, I mean for a while, and then they stop eventually.

Therapist: What are the worries about these thoughts, and what would happen if you did give them some space, to stop fighting with them?

Susie: I don't know, I can just see that they would be so overwhelming, and then, well, it makes it more real. I don't want to think about the end. And I don't want to picture those horrible things.

Therapist: Like somehow giving it space will mean that these things happen?

Susie: (Quietly) Maybe. Like somehow it is more real if I give into it.

Therapist: That's a scary thought, right? And I can see why your brain is trying to help you by thinking that if you don't think about it, then it can't be real. The only problem is that it is showing up anyway – you work really hard during the day for these thoughts not to show up, and then they just come at night when you aren't able to work so hard to fight with them.

Susie: Maybe.

Therapist: Can I give you a strange example? Do you remember as a kid doing a tug of war?[1]

Susie: Yeah.

Therapist: So, right now, you are in a tug of war with these thoughts/emotions/worries and anything else that might be showing up about the future. These worries are showing up because of this health stuff, and we know that they are showing up about the important things – the kids, the future, what means a lot to you. And, we wouldn't want to get rid of that – because those things are important.

Susie: Right.

Therapist: So what is your instinct when you are in a tug of war?

Susie: You keep pulling as hard as you can, until you beat the other team.

Therapist: That's what most of us do. We keep fighting and fighting. But you know what, these things across from you – they aren't going to go away. You have tried so hard to get rid of them, and you are exhausted from trying. And they are standing there ready to keep going – the grief, the sadness, the worry, the anger and the hurt, and probably a million more. Just ready to fight some more.

Susie: So, what do I do then?

Therapist: You drop the rope.

Susie: I drop the rope?

Therapist: Yup. Nothing changes with those thoughts. Those worries and thoughts are still there, and you could start that fight to get rid of them again whenever you want. But if we know that they aren't going to get rid of them, and that they have a job. But, if you aren't fighting with them all of the time, and you can make friends with them, it allows you more space to do all the other stuff.

Susie: That's great, but what does that actually mean?

Therapist: It means when those thoughts and worries show up, you recognise them for what they are. You might have a conversation with your mind to say – 'Ah, grief, there you are. I see you. I know that you are trying to help me'. But the thing that changes is that you aren't then fighting with everything to get rid of it.

We are going to continue this conversation with Susie when we move on to the defusion/thought management section. You will notice again, that just like values and committed action, over the course of the session/discussion, you may move around various pieces of the hexaflex, and visit/revisit concepts that you have explored before.

Troubleshooting Acceptance

As we have named multiple times throughout the book, one of the biggest challenges that you will come across when working with acceptance is likely to be the complexity of identifying that we are not asking people to accept the 'death' (or other hard things that are showing up), but rather the emotion around it. This sounds simple but is territory that will need to be navigated over and over again.

◆ Therapist frustration may show up here around the ideas of having to revisit different aspects of people's experiences and patients struggling to connect across domains. This is more likely to occur with people at end of life when their disease process, pain or medications impact on their capacity to be cognitively flexible and abstract. This isn't fixable necessarily but can be helpful to notice in your own practice.

◆ Sometimes there is a natural limit to the acceptance space – where you have been able to name the emotion, notice its presence, and make space for it, but the person will continue to struggle and have difficulty engaging around it. Again, this is often a process of the situation and the complexity. In this space it is helpful to model and be curious about the acceptance role, but also be flexible in practice to the ways that this might be showing up. Sometimes even with openness and acceptance things can feel stuck.

◆ It can also be important to identify if a patient is misplacing the idea of acceptance of emotion to becoming resigned to a situation. If you are noticing that this is happening, or there is confusion in the room, it is important to revisit the ideas around acceptance and openness.

Note

1 The Tug of War metaphor is very common within ACT practice. A further explanation can be found in *The Happiness Trap* (Harris, 2021).

15

Present Focus (Including When the Present Is Really Hard!)

In the context of unknowness and uncertainty facing most people who are approaching end of life, the role of being able to connect with the present moment is particularly important. As we have discussed earlier, most people will experience anxiety, for some people this may be the first time that they have experienced anxious worries or ruminations. It may also be one of the first times that people have experienced a situation where problem solving and behavioural strategies do not provide relief.

There has been a significant explosion of ideas around mindfulness and present focus in the last couple of years – so it is unlikely that the ideas will be completely foreign to the people that you are seeing. However, it may be that they have significant ideas about what it means to be mindful, and may have tried strategies that have not been what they expected. I am often careful to not use the words, like mindfulness or particularly meditation, where people may have these pre-conceptions, instead using phrasing like 'connecting with the here and now' or 'being in the moment' or simply about 'being present'.

Many people will assume the role of present-focused work is to remove the presence of anxiety or any difficulties that they are experiencing. It is important (as with all ACT components)

DOI: 10.4324/9781003431640-18

to reiterate that the goal of any work around the present focus is not about the removal of discomfort or anxiety, instead it is about making space and allowing connection with what is important.

The other important consideration is in thinking about the capacity that people who are unwell will have around present-focused practice. In my experience, and what many of my colleagues in this space have reported, is that despite good intentions around wanting to do 'mindfulness' activities their fidelity around regular practice and engagement is usually limited. Any activities or practice that you recommend will likely need to be simple, readily available and quick. There of course will be exceptions to this rule, and on occasion I have met people who have had strong mindfulness practice prior to diagnosis who are able to maintain and build on it when unwell – but they are very much the exception.

Framing of Present Focus

It is important that you are clear about the utility of present focus practice. Thinking about the conceptions that people may bring to this space, if you don't communicate well, or explain why the role of present focus is important you will likely lose them. It sounds simple, but it is one of the areas of ACT that in my experience people *under* explain compared with the other areas where we tend to *over* explain.

There are lots of ways to do this, but generally I have found something along the lines of:

> It sounds like much of what you are worried about is future based – all the uncertainty, the anxiety and those worries about what is going to happen next. And of course, those worries are trying to help you and have a purpose, but I wonder what happens when you are in the moment rather than when you are getting swept up in the future stuff.

Some people may not need further prompts and will be able to connect with this concept easily. Others may require more prompting, such as:

> I wonder if you can think about a time where you are just in the moment and not thinking about other things. For lots of people, this might be when they are out in the sunshine and listening to the birds, or just watching people go about their days. You know the things that just grab us and pull our attention.

Usually after such a prompt they will be better able to identify things where this is the case. This then allows an exploration of what happens for them in those moments where they are present, and noticing what happens to the thoughts. Some helpful questions might be:

◆ What happens in those moments when you are just present to what is happening in the here and now? What do you notice about how you feel?
◆ Are there times when you notice that you can connect with the present more than others? What's different about these times?
◆ What happens to time when you are swept up in your thoughts?
◆ What feels different between the times when you are present and when you get caught in the thoughts?

Usually, exploring these concepts will allow people to connect and engage with why present-focus practice is helpful.

When the Present Is Really Hard

There is a reality about end of life that is important to consider when we are exploring present focus. For many people that you will work with in this space, the current moment will be challenging in itself. And the next moment might also be hard. And for some people, the idea of bringing their attention and focus to the present is going to feel completely inconceivable. They may be spending all of their time doing everything that they can to not be present – and it may be that they are experiencing the worst of two worlds. They may be avoiding being present because of the hardness, whilst ruminating about the uncertain future and anticipating the ways in which it is worse than it is now. For people where this is the case, it is important to explore what is happening for them – what are the thoughts that are arising, but also, what are their thoughts about the thoughts and the utility of how this shows up. It may be, that at these times (particularly when very unwell or in significant pain), trying to connect with the current moment will be much less helpful than distraction or other things that the patient has come up with.

The ideas around escape fantasies may be showing up here as well – where they are focusing on some alternative view of the future – which allows some sense of agency or control. This can be the times when passive suicidal ideation may arise, or focus or fixation on alternative endings (where doing a particular thing will change everything). Most of the time when these things are occurring gentle exploration will be helpful to identify what the drivers of these thoughts may be, as well as their utility.

In these moments of hardness – it is important to focus on process rather than outcome. The goal of the present focus isn't about getting rid of the hardness – instead it is about thinking about the role that being present and connected plays in how they want to be in the world.

There may be genuine times where being connected to the present is not helpful. An example of this may be when people are in significant pain or having particular physical symptoms. Occasionally there may be helpfulness in bringing awareness and attention to these experiences, but for most patients this will not be the case. Instead, they will likely actively work to do things that cognitively distract them from the pain. It would be very difficult to shift people from this space in those moments in time, and actually remaining disconnected from such significant pain is protective.

It can be helpful to emphasise that the goal isn't to be present all the time. No one can manage this, but many patients will interpret that the measure of success is to be present 100% of the time (particularly in the context of being unwell). For those people who are very unwell, or in pain, it may be helpful to help them navigate to even very brief instances of present-moment connection – such as noticing the feel of the sun on their skin, or a snippet of conversation.

Simple Present Focus Strategies

Almost all practitioners will have their own go-to strategies that they have found good language and comfort in using. If you have some of these that work well, then I would encourage you to continue to use them, perhaps making small changes to make them more suitable to use when people are physically unwell or have limited capacity.

There are a couple of categories of strategies that are staples in working in this space:

◆ Bringing awareness to the body.
◆ Bringing awareness to thoughts and emotions.
◆ Bringing awareness to the external environment.
◆ Bringing awareness to the imagination.

Bringing Awareness to the Body
Of the three categories of present-focused work, this is the one which is least likely to be helpful with those who are unwell. As mentioned above, for some they will be able to do work to connect with the physical sensations that are present, however for most people when physically very unwell, connecting with these will likely cause significant distress. Most patients will likely be hyper-aware of the physical symptoms and so drawing further attention will likely be counterproductive. The same applies to using breathing-focused exercises in those who are experiencing lung concerns or having changes in breathing.

In the absence of any of the above, the best exercises in my experience have been things like:

1. Intentional breathing – asking the person to bring attention to the speed of their breathing (not about depth or effectiveness of the breath). Asking to breathe in for three seconds (one thousand, two thousand, three thousand) and then out for three seconds (four thousand, five thousand, six thousand). Repeat this 10 times.
2. Counting breaths – asking the person to count the breaths that they take in a minute. Can do this by setting a timer on their phone and counting them. Let them know that the lower the number the better.
3. General body scan – systematically bringing awareness to each part of their body. If the person has an isolated physical symptom this can still work very well, I would just not bring attention to that particular part of their body, or ask that they focus on a different part instead if they are doing a version of this exercise at home.
4. Isolated body awareness – asking them to bring awareness to a particular body part or particular body movement. For instance, being aware of the sensation of rubbing their feet together under a quilt, examining their hand or noticing the sensation of pushing their feet into the floor. These can work well, even when someone is unwell, as it requires relatively little energy.

Bringing Awareness to Thoughts and Emotions

As above, someone's ability to engage in these activities is very contingent on how well they are. However, simple exercises that bring attention to the person's experience of their thoughts can be particularly helpful in the acceptance work that we spoke about in the last chapter. It can also help them identify when thoughts are showing up – this may sound simple enough, but for many people who are experiencing such significant experiences of thoughts and emotions (that they likely haven't encountered before) it can be very helpful to bring a present focus to this.

Some suggested strategies:

1. Watching their thoughts – this can be a variation on the Leaves on the Stream exercises that are very common ACT practice, or doing some prompted and guided discussion with the person around noticing their thoughts when they arise. Asking questions such as – do the thoughts turn up as words or as pictures? Do they flash across all at once, or are they more like a story, how do the thoughts move from one to another?

Bringing Awareness to the External Environment

This group of exercises includes ones that most people can identify with and connect to. Part of the appeal of these is the simplicity, but also the low energy component. In addition, it allows people to focus on something outside of themselves, which, when people are unwell, can be a significant challenge.

Some exercises are as follows:

1. Engaging the senses – using hearing is a good one, but can use all five (again, be aware that people have particular physical concerns – you would likely avoid using taste and smell in those patients with particular head and neck conditions, or on treatments that impair their functioning in those areas). Ask the person to come up with five things that they can connect to right now (What can they hear? What can they see? etc.). This exercise is quite quick, but most people will identify the connection to the present.

2. Noticing what is happening around them. If they are able to go and sit outside, ask them to pay attention to what nature is happening around them (birds, insects, their pets). They need to really pay attention – what are they doing? What are they going to do next? What does their facial expression tell them? Don't underestimate

how powerful the connection to nature is when people are in existential distress!

3. Noticing sensations – if they are able to get outside, ask them to notice the feeling of the sun on their shoulders, or the wind on their face. If they aren't able to get outside, Ask them to notice the way the light changes in the house/room during the day.

4. Tuning into external things – this works well for people who are very immobile and perhaps can't change their environment easily. When listening to music (or another consistent sound) ask them to tune into one particular element – drums work particularly well. Ask them to try and focus only on the drums and the sound that they are making.

Bringing Awareness to the Imagination

These strategies do not work for everyone, but can be powerful in those who are able to easily visualise things (I would ask them before suggesting these!) or for those who are very unwell. Many patients will describe a version of these exercises when they are unwell, or unable to mobilise where they find their mind picturing and creating things for them. Some of these are not present-focused activities per se, but will allow them to focus on the experience of the memory, rather than ruminations or other experiences that they are having.

1. *Visualise something* – these mindfulness exercises are very powerful in children and young people, but I have found that adults can also find them helpful. I would encourage them to listen to a guided prompt (readily available) for something that resonates with them – going to the beach, walking in a garden, going on a holiday, etc.

2. *Replay a favourite movie* – Ask them to think of their favourite TV show or movie and play the first five minutes back in their minds. This sounds like it will be very simple, but many of us struggle to do this, as our brain will jump ahead on us!

3. *Replay a memory* – ask them to think about a favourite memory and to replay it. Make sure that you emphasise the need for detail and give them some prompts as needed. What was the weather like? What were you wearing? What was one thing that you noticed in that moment? What was around you? What could you smell?

I am certain that there are thousands of other exercises that I haven't recommended here – and there will be a bunch of people who read this and think, I would never do those! That's ok! It is important that you find a good language and tone for the exercises that you are asking people to do. I would also never ask anyone to do anything that I haven't done or tried. Give these (and any others) a go and see how they feel – if they don't land with you, it's a reasonable chance that you won't be able to describe them or convince someone else that they will work.

Noticing the Small Things (Bringing Gratitude)

Including this in this space is likely to be a bit controversial, however, many of my patients have reported that engaging in gratitude practice can be a key component of their present-focused engagement, and particularly those at end of life have found it helpful.

The main ways that I have seen people engage with grati-tude practice at end of life is very similar to many of the other strategies that we have spoken about so far in this chapter – they are based around processes of routine, simplicity, and requiring low energy. Although some will find journalling and writing about gratitude a helpful process, for most it will be much more informal (and at times incidental).

A good suggestion for practice is to notice a couple of things per day that they feel grateful for or connected to. There is importance in the setup of this, and it is key to make sure that you are clear about the role of gratitude, and being explicit that it isn't about making them feel okay about their situation. It might be helpful to frame the use of gratitude practice in the context of connecting with present, and being aware of the things that help make their world rich if people are struggling with this. I might frame it something like this:

> It's funny, when things aren't feeling great in our worlds we can get caught up in the terrible, but there are usually a bunch of things, mostly quite small stuff that actually makes our world rich despite all the hard. Lots of my patients find connecting with these small things helpful, and they find that coming up with a few things each day will allow them to be present to it. For example, I spoke with someone earlier in the week, and in noticing the birds singing outside the window each morning, they also noticed that they felt grateful about being able to witness them, and that they were able to connect with them. Nothing has changed – the person is still there, the bird is still singing, but they were then tuned into how much they were glad that they could hear it in that moment.

This will resonate with some people much more than others, and so if it doesn't land with someone, that is completely okay.

Troubleshooting Present Focus

Present focus when working with people in this space can be inherently difficult.

◆ It is important to reinforce here that present focus can show up in a difficult way in two ways, which are in different directions – it can be almost impossible for people to connect with (because their brain is spinning into the future where the present is too hard) or it can be all that people focus on (particularly if they are unwell or in pain – in which case, distraction is a better tool). When this occurs it is helpful to name it, and allow the person to connect with the reality of why it is hard for them to show up in the present.

◆ If you are finding that the person you are working with is getting caught up in the *idea* of present-focus work rather than the actual work, it can be important to reframe the purpose of doing the work, or even rename it to help them disconnect from the thinking about the process.

◆ You may notice that for many people the burden of feeling that they need to do 'another thing' can get in the way of their practice. This can be particularly true around ideas of meditation and mindfulness, where it is likely that many people are telling them to do it. It will likely not be helpful to be seen as getting caught up in this, and so it is probably worth pausing the work, reframing and setting realistic sets of expectations (which might be not to do anything outside of a session).

◆ If the ideas of present focus aren't resonating with someone, move on. It may be that it isn't the right time, or that they don't have capacity.

16

Thought Management and Defusion

Doing cognitive work with people at end of life is likely to present challenges that look quite different from doing this work in other populations. Firstly, as we have spoken about over and over again throughout the book, how well someone is physically will have a very significant impact on how able they are to engage in strictly cognitive work. Now of course, ACT looks quite different from other modalities where there are distinct activities or exercises that are more cognitively focused vs behaviourally based – and so if the person is unable to engage in cognitive work the focus may shift to a more behavioural model. However, as we have discovered as we have moved around the hexaflex, within ACT this is much less defined, and a common session is likely to mean moving around a little between domains on the hexaflex. The work around defusion that we are going to describe here is quite experiential and will focus on simple concepts. You may have existing strategies that work well, and if this is the case, I would encourage you to use them (albeit with some amendments around the thoughts/processes specific to end of life).

Secondly, for most of the people you will meet their thoughts will have two characteristics. Those fears and worries that people are describing, will for the most part be similar in character to others that you will have encountered elsewhere – the defining difference is that the worries are likely to be based firmly in

DOI: 10.4324/9781003431640-19

reality. People will describe thoughts about suffering, death, catastrophic situations, pain and imagine their own coping. It is incredibly difficult to sit in a space with someone, with these thoughts and to recognise their reality. This is the time when clinicians will most often tap into their own sense of helplessness and start to panic (usually by throwing strategies and suggestions at people). We will talk more about this in the next section, but it is important to check in with yourself during these times to make sure that the work that you are doing remains consistent and not getting diluted by throwing strategies into the mix (this tends to cause confusion for the client and the therapist!). The second characteristic is that there is likely to be difficult emotions and thoughts that show up. These are the ones that are hardest for us all to sit with – things like guilt, shame, regret. As people approach the end of life, the things that they are talking with you about are likely to be the really tricky ones, and it is important to recognise this both for the patient, but also for yourself as you navigate through this.

Thinking in Itself

I often reflect that regular people – i.e., those who don't spend their lives thinking about thinking – don't think about thoughts in the way that therapists do. We learn very early on in our training to recognize the errant ideas and concepts that arrive in peoples' brains, and we work out what to do with them (even if that thing is acceptance). For most people you will encounter, though, not only will they not have thought about the way they think, they will have no reason to question the content or reality of those thoughts. So when we are talking about something as salient as the approach to the end of life, where the thoughts feel very real, but the consequences of those thoughts feel equally real, it is much more challenging to work with people around this.

Although I am sure that everyone who is reading this is going to be very tuned into the impact that they can have on people when we start talking about thoughts – particularly around invalidation, it bears repeating that we need to be very cautious when dealing with content of thoughts to not get into the challenging of content, but also on the flip side, not invalidating the things that are coming up for people.

It is important to pause with people and recognize the process of thinking about what is happening for them, before moving on to other strategies and techniques. This can be something quite simple, but is aimed at bringing their awareness to what is happening in their minds.

It might be something like:

It sounds like there is a lot of thoughts flying around in your mind at the moment. I wonder if it might be helpful for us to get to know some of those better?

Or

It's funny how these thoughts seems to arrive whenever you aren't busy doing other things. I wonder what is happening in that? What is happening when they aren't showing up versus when they are?

Or

How are these things showing up for you? For some people these thoughts are words, or pictures, or they might even sound like voices. How is it to be in your brain at the moment?

Or

What's your headspace like at the moment? Is there much chatter in there about what is going on?

Now, of course, you will need to find your own prompting questions that fits with your style, but most people will respond well to the versions of the above.

Sometimes, people will be in such a strong space of avoidance that it might be hard to tap into their internal experience –

particularly in the context of thoughts about death and dying. If this is the case, and gentle prompts are not effective, it can be better to change tack and explore other aspects, and then circle back to the more difficult thoughts at a later time when they are feeling more able to approach them. We know that the people who are coming to speak to a therapist are the ones who are willing to talk about things, but many of the thoughts that they are having might be things that they have never put language too (and like we spoke about earlier, it might feel like putting language to them will in some way make something bad happen).

Getting Space

Its likely that simple explanations will be best around the ideas of defusion. The way that I would normally describe this will be around 'getting space'.

There are a bunch of awesome experiential strategies that you can use to describe this process (I won't describe these here, but are readily available in most ACT resources). The one that seems to resonate particularly well with people is using your hand to demonstrate distance.

Using the hand as a prompt can be a very helpful way of not only demonstrating the concept of space as it is likely that this isn't a concept that people will have thought about before, but also allows a visual representation of how much room the thoughts are taking up – again something the people may not have thought about.

Therapist: It sounds like these thoughts are pretty loud and taking lots of energy.

Client: Yeah, I just can't turn them off.

Therapist: I am not sure that it is about turning them off.

Client: What do you mean?

Therapist: I think these thoughts are coming because of the situation that you are in. It makes sense that these worries are showing up. But it sounds like at the moment they are right here (holds up hand so that it is covering the therapist's face), and I wonder if we might be able to think about how we get a bit more space in there so that you have a bit more room to think about where you are, but also for other things (moves hand away from the face). I don't think we will get rid of them, but getting some more room and space will probably help.

Client: (Nods) It would be good to have a break from them.

Therapist: I wonder if we might be able to do some work to help you recognise what is happening when they show up which might help a bit with getting a little bit of time where you aren't so connected to them.

It is then much easier to move into conversation about acceptance, other defusion strategies and any other cognitive work.

This may also be an opportunity to combine a more formal defusion strategy like 'I am having the thought that' with the intention of reinforcing the cognitive component of getting distance from the thoughts. Given the content of the thoughts it is important to use any strategies carefully as it may be easy for patients to misinterpret the defusion strategies as invalidating the reality of the thoughts.

As we discussed in the chapter on acceptance, you may need to revisit multiple times the idea of making space, room and allowing the presence of thoughts – and that getting rid of them is not the goal. Some people will be able to make sense of this easily, where others will continue to revisit the goal of being free of the thoughts and worries. For these people, this work will likely be incremental, but by remaining consistent in your approach and modelling acceptance in session it will allow reference points for the client to draw from.

When Thoughts Are Just Thoughts

With the salience of thoughts about end of life, it will be challenging for patients to recognise that the thoughts are just thoughts. This is quite different from when working with very

anxious or depressed patients who may be able to readily recognise the cognitive component of what is happening for them.
You may need to do substantial work with people around recognising the disparity between what they are thinking and the
reality of it.

Client: And then when I have the treatment it is going to
make me feel terrible and then it starts, doesn't it?
Stuck in bed and not being able to look after the kids.
What kind of a mother am I?

Therapist: I don't know whether you noticed this, but it feels
like you just moved very quickly to how terrible
things are going to be.

Client: But that's what chemo does. When I had treatment
before, I ended up in bed for days each cycle. So I
need to be prepared.

Therapist: I totally get that, the stakes are high here (pause). We
talked lots about how hard it was for you to not be
able to turn up the way that you wanted, and I can see
why your brain is trying to plan for if that were to
happen again. But, I wonder if we might not be
getting caught up in the thoughts about what might
happen instead of what is actually happening.

Client: What do you mean?

Therapist: Well, I wonder what you know for sure about this
treatment right now?

Client: Well the oncologist said that it won't be too bad, but
he has been wrong before, and he isn't the one who
has to have it and be sick.

Therapist: No, he doesn't. But it strikes me that right here and
right now, you are intending to do the treatment.[1]

Client: Well, of course. I would do anything.

Therapist: So, I guess I would like us to better understand how
much your brain is filling in for you – particularly
around the stuff about how terrible it is going to be.

Client: Probably a lot.

Therapist: And it's doing that to be helpful. But, I think maybe
it isn't being that helpful. It sounds like getting

	caught up in thoughts is keeping you awake at night and leaving you feeling pretty panicked and anxious about the future.
Client:	Well, that's true. But I can't stop it.
Therapist:	I think in thinking about stopping it we are getting pulled into the detail, but I wonder whether it might be helpful to tease out what we know for sure, rather what our brain is filling in.
Client:	And how do I do that?
Therapist:	That's a good question. I wonder if it isn't a simple answer – but maybe the first step is getting to know these thoughts a little better. Maybe a helpful question to help tease it out might be 'what do I know right now for sure?'
Client:	So that I can get rid of the other stuff?
Therapist:	I wonder if a better question might not be about thinking of 'how do we manage the thoughts better so that you have some more space'?
Client:	Mmmm. I know that you say that they won't go – but if I could just know that the treatment isn't going to make me sick like the last time, then I would be fine.
Therapist:	Mmm, that's interesting, isn't it? I wonder though whether that is the certainty story that we have talked about before showing up – if you could change one thing, that everything would be better.
Client:	Oh. I didn't even catch that.
Therapist:	Our brains are pretty sneaky sometimes. (Pauses) I don't think we will get rid of it, but I wonder if with some more space it might mean that you have a bit more capacity for the things that we know are really important.

Once the person has an improved awareness of the way that thoughts are not reality, it will allow you to work with them in a way to help increase cognitive flexibility around how these thoughts are not only showing up, but how they are impacting in the day to day.

Naming and Externalising Thoughts

It can be particularly complex for people in this space to
separate out thoughts/emotions/physical experiences. In recognising this, it may be helpful to provide prompts, language
and models to help them become familiar with their internal
processes.

One of the best ways to do this is to help them name and
separate out the 'characters' of the emotions/thoughts that are
showing up. This can also be helpful in recognising the stories
that are arising (although it is important to note that when
naming stories it is to do so judiciously and sparingly as to not
risk invalidation).

As an example, this has been a helpful tool in working with
a patient of mine around grief.

Therapist: I might be wrong about this, and please tell me if I
am, but it sounds like the grief is turning up in lots of
places at the moment.

Client: (Nods and becomes teary)

Therapist: I don't think we have named it like that before,
have we?

Client: No. I think we have talked about bits of it, but I don't
think I have ever thought about it as grief.

Therapist: What do you notice about naming it?

Client: (Pauses) Um, I don't know really. It feels more
reasonable somehow.

Therapist: What do you mean by that?

Client: Um. Well, it is, isn't it, I am grieving for knowing
that I am going, but I think it has been showing up
and I haven't noticed it. Well, I haven't noticed it as
grief.

Therapist: How do you think you have been seeing it?

Client: I think I have been focusing on each thing. The
frustration or the sadness, without stepping back
from it to see the grief.

Therapist: And what do you see with it, when you can take
those steps back?

Client: I can see a bit more about how I have been responding in a really emotional way, and sometimes that I haven't been as rational as I would like to be.

Therapist: (Laughs gently) I don't know that grief shows up in a very rational way.

Client: (Laughs) That's true.

Therapist: But, I would imagine that there is a predictability about the story that the grief gives.

Client: I think that now that I think about it – it is mostly that it is showing up around the future and worry. Every time I think about what might happen, there is all of this other stuff that shows up too. I hadn't thought about this being grief before.

Therapist: I sometimes think of those characters that live in our brain – we have thousands of them. And for you, it sounds like that grief guy is sitting on your shoulder at the moment and being pretty loud for everything that shows up.

Client: I think so. He definitely has a lot to say. (Laughs)

Therapist: I wonder if it might be worth trying to notice and catch it when that guy is showing up. It sounds like thinking about this stuff as grief is helpful and so, if you can identify it whenever it shows, I wonder what might look different.

Client: It already feels less big somehow.

Therapist: Like how?

Client: Like now that I can see it, it doesn't quite have the same pull.

Therapist: That's pretty powerful, isn't it? And nothing has changed. Those thoughts and emotions are still showing up, and I think they will keep doing it.

Client: I think that might be part of it, though – I think I have been fighting to make it disappear, but then when they don't, I am getting frustrated and sad.

Therapist: So maybe part of recognising the grief guy is recognising that he is always going to be there. Sometimes he might be quiet, and sometimes he might be screaming in your ear, but the consistency

	is that he will show up.
Client:	Like that annoying neighbour that lives down the end of the street. (laughs)
Therapist:	(laughs). Even more persistent likely. (Pauses) But that's part of it as well. When he shows up, there is almost a part of it 'Ah! Grief, I have been expecting you!'
Client:	At least it is predictable.
Therapist:	I wonder whether this grief is a much a part of treatment as the chemo and the pain meds. It is what shows up for you in the face of this tricky stuff.
Client:	I hadn't thought about it like that.

Once you have named the presence and externalised one of these emotions/thoughts, it is much easier to then generalise across multiple domains for the person. Furthermore, having named them, it allows you to do a shortcut of sorts in therapy as well, being able to reflect back and 'name' the emotions/thoughts when they show up.

Trouble Shooting Defusion

It goes without saying that defusion in this population group is a delicate process. Many of the thoughts/worries/emotions that you will encounter in this context are not only appropriate but adaptive, and so it is important to ensure that the defusion work is not invalidating (even unintentionally).

◆ As above, use formal defusion strategies to get distance and demonstrate the same sparingly. If you try something and it doesn't land, ensure that you revisit with the patient what your intention is in doing the defusion work is.

◆ Some people will not have the capacity for defusion when they are unwell, in pain, or cognitively impacted in any way. If you notice that your patient is struggling, it is okay to focus on processes that are more immediate and require less cognitive work.

◆ Even for the most committed patient, you may find that the work done in session doesn't translate to change between sessions – this is very common in this group where the levels of task loading is significant. You may find that writing things down, or using very metaphor-heavy examples will help, but there may be a reality that there is less capacity for them to do this work on this space (particularly when unwell).

◆ It is important to reinforce that the process of defusion is ongoing – they will need to continue to be present for, and to practice this many many times, and in different contexts. Defusion isn't a helpful intervention, just for the sake of defusion, and so it is important to revisit regularly how the function of defusion is helping to facilitate the things that are important to the patient.

Note

1 This conversation can go in a couple of directions from here – we can keep focusing on the thoughts, or could move to a space around decision making. In the chapter on problem solving, we explore the ways that exploring decision making can look.

17

Self as Context

Of all of the aspects of ACT, self as context is the one that is likely to puzzle people the most. There are few reasons for this, not the least of which is that it is hard for therapists to grasp conceptually, which in turn means that it is particularly difficult to translate this for the people that we see. There are many analogies and metaphors that help demonstrate this, but within the end of life context, I suspect that it will be quite difficult to apply these.

The process of self as context is about being able to recognize the parts of ourself which is outside of our thoughts/cognitions and emotions. However, if we again revisit the idea of how people think about their thinking – for most people when unwell they will struggle to separate out the thoughts as separate from their physical and somatic experience, and so to extend this to become aware of the process of observing their thinking this will feel quite nebulous and out of reach.

It is likely that if you get caught up in trying to describe the process of self as context the patient will likely get lost, and so, it is helpful to find ways to give examples of how this is showing up in their lives and to help them apply. Luckily, ACT is all about the experiential aspects!

I have described some of the strategies that work well within this space, however, if you have other metaphors/ideas that you have found to work I would encourage you to try amending these for this population!

DOI: 10.4324/9781003431640-20

If I Were Watching You ...

Like many of the concepts that we have discussed, some of the best ways to introduce patients to the concepts that we are discussing is to model them in the therapeutic conversation to help give insight and awareness to make sense of what is playing out. One of the best ways to do this is to explore what an external person watching them would observe. This process allows several processes to occur at once. Firstly, it does some work around defusion and getting some distance and space from the experience of what is happening, but secondly, it allows them to have a sense of perspective outside of themselves. This is quite similar to the psychotherapeutic questioning around perspective taking – allowing the person to step outside their own experience to understand how it might be for others, but in this instance the focus is on what is happening in their mind and how that is playing out.

Some of the questions that serve as helpful prompts around this might be things like:

If I were watching a movie of what is happening for you, what would I see?

Or

If I were a fly on the wall watching what is happening in your brain, what would I see?

Or

If you had to describe these characters that are showing up in your mind, how would they be?

A nice conversation that I had with a patient this week around grief highlighted the way that simple analogies and metaphors can work well. We were talking about her reflections of the grief of her situation, as we spoke about the transition from content to context.

Patient: It's funny. It's been a year since all of this started, and I was looking back on it, and I just realised that this grief exists just as it is.

Therapist: This sounds interesting. What do you mean?

Patient: Well, last year, I think I was so caught up in it, and all of the emotions, it was hard to see anything. But now, I can see that this is just the place that I am – there was a place before, and maybe there is a place after, but ...

Therapist: This might sound strange, but it reminds me a bit of a pool.

Patient: A pool?

Therapist: Yeah. So when all of this first happened, you are just in the water in the grief, swimming around and struggling to work out how to get out. And then a little while ago you noticed that you were better able to notice when the grief was present – where you are standing on the edge of the pool and looking at the grief. But now it sounds like you are on the high board looking down on the grief – you can see that it has a start and end point, and that there is space outside of it. That doesn't mean that you don't ever go swimming again, but it feels like for now at least it's easier to see it for what it is.

The response that people have to these prompts will usually lead to the opportunity to have further exploration about the ways that they think about their thoughts, the relationship to the thoughts, and the ways that they are making sense of how they are showing up. If you feel that you are hitting resistance with this, it might be helpful to explore some of the other strategies we have discussed (particularly when looking at acceptance and thought defusion) to get people more familiar with their cognitions to then try and observe them in a different way. In my experience, if you jump to self as context too early people will get quite lost in the complexity of it, and miss what you are trying to do – which is ultimately about increasing cognitive flexibility around their thoughts and thinking.

Thinking About Thinking

Another useful tool to use from a self as context perspective is the idea of making people more aware of the process of thinking about their thinking. If we approach this in a practical example, it can be a reasonably easy way for people to conceptualise this. This also serves a dual purpose around getting some space in how people are recognizing thoughts, but also in recognizing patterns of how they respond when difficult experiences/emotions show up. The important component in this is to help people recognise that despite the situation (which may be fixed or even deteriorating) the thoughts around the situation/emotions are not fixed.

A really simple example of this is something that comes up in people at end of life frequently. Most people will experience some level of sleep disturbance – either as a result of physical experiences or ruminations/worries.

Therapist: So, tell me about what is happening with your sleep.

Client: It's horrible. I get off to sleep, and then I wake about midnight, uncomfortable and in pain, and I toss and turn for hours trying to get back to sleep.

Therapist: So, what is happening in those hours of tossing and turning.

Client: I am thinking, and then getting really frustrated. Often I am getting really distressed about not being able to sleep. I know that to have the best chance of survival I have to do all these things – good diet, sleep and exercise. So, then if I am not sleeping, I start to think about how I am doing the worst thing that I could be doing, and if I could just get to sleep I would be able to work towards cure. I get angry and frustrated at my body. And then I get angry and frustrated at myself. More than anything I just want to turn off the thoughts so that I can sleep.

Therapist: Wow. That is a lot of pressure to put on sleeping.

Client: Yeah, it is. It feels quite overwhelming actually.

Therapist: I bet. And my guess is that thinking about all of that doesn't make getting to sleep any easier?

Client: It doesn't. Instead, I just get really caught up in the thoughts, and then I start to panic.

Therapist: So, in lots of ways it isn't the not sleeping that is the problem, it is all of the stuff that comes along with the not sleeping …

Client: Well, the not sleeping means that my cancer might get worse.

Therapist: I can see that this is a really tricky thing for you to manage – the stakes feel really high, and so then there is a bunch of stuff that turns up around it. I wonder whether it is not the sleeping that is really the problem here?

Client: What do you mean?

Therapist: Well, I think it is actually the thinking about the sleeping, and then even the thinking about the thinking about the sleeping that is getting in the way more.

Client: I don't understand.

Therapist: Well, my sense, and tell me if I am wrong, but it sounds like there is something that is pretty concrete happening with your sleep – you are waking up with physical discomfort or something else. So that is the thing itself – the not sleeping. But then your brain is showing up, and having all of these thoughts about not sleeping – the things like 'The cancer is going to get worse because I am not sleeping'. And then the thoughts about the thoughts about not sleeping show up – the ones where the blame shows up about how if you were sleeping than the cancer would be okay and if it isn't, it is somehow your fault. And I am guessing it would go on and on from there?

Client: Yeah, I guess.

Therapist: So, I am not sure that we can do anything necessarily about the not sleeping – it sounds like that is out of your control, particularly the physical stuff. It sounds like you are going to wake up, or you aren't, and that isn't anything that you can do something about. But, I am wondering if recognizing those thoughts and worries, and then the thinking about those thoughts and worries might be the thing that we can work on together.

You can use this approach in almost anything where there are cognitions turning up about an experience itself. I often find myself saying to patients that the 'anxiety itself isn't a problem. It is unpleasant, sure, and nobody wants to be anxious, but we as humans are meant to be anxious at times. What is more difficult to manage by the sound of it are the thoughts and worries about how the anxiety will show up, or panicking about the anxiety showing up.'

By approaching it in this way, not only do you have the opportunity to start to work with the acceptance of the thoughts turning up, but also in doing some concrete strategies to address the underlying concerns (this applies particularly well to sleep, but would be just as apt if working with anxiety, low mood or relationship concerns). It is important to recognise that this is not a pure self-as-context intervention – but can be a helpful tool when working with people around the awareness and changeability of the thoughts that arise in the context of difficult physical experiences.

Working With the Sense of Self

For the people that we are working with at end of life – they are going to be in a state of flux, with considerable uncertainty about the future, but also considerable changes and impacts about how they are showing up in the here and now. For many people, the things that have gone alongside their illness will mean that much of the core 'essence' of them will feel like it has been stripped away. In ACT practice, there are concepts around the transcendent self, and the stable sense of self (I won't go into detail about this here, but is good background reading If needed is available in many ACT textbooks and resources listed at the back of the book). Simply, the stable sense of self is the piece of us which is unchanged despite many challenging things happening around us, or to our worlds. An extension of this is the idea of the transcendent self which is the piece that is about recognizing the pieces of you that never change even in the face of constant change.

For many patients at end of life, these will be difficult concepts to access, however, the concepts of sense of self can be a helpful conversation and work to explore, particularly in those who are struggling in the context of change, and having significant things taken from them. It can be particularly powerful to explore what remains constant and unchanged.

Some of the prompts around this might be:

In the face of everything that is moving and shifting, which are the parts of you, particularly in your mind, that remain unchanged?

Or

When you think about everything that is going on, is there something that you are always able to go back to?

This will definitely not be for most patients, but for a select few, these conversations can be particularly powerful, and will often result in a deep existential discussion.

Trouble Shooting Self as Context

Self as context can be difficult to conceptualise, particularly if you think too much about it. The most important thing when embarking on this work is to recognise that it isn't a stand alone intervention.

◆ Self as context is a powerful tool in helping people at end of life recognise the roles that they hold, and how they are thinking about their disease process.

◆ Simplicity is the key. If you get too complex people will get lost! If they are struggling, slow down, link the self as context back to what you are working with (might be defusion, values or acceptance) and try reframing. If you are still feeling stuck, leave it and come back to revisit later. If it's important it will surface again.

◆ Self as context more than anything requires a good conceptual understanding before trying to explain this to patients (otherwise it will get very confusing very quickly!) It can be helpful to try and out some of the metaphors and descriptions to help you make sense of it for yourself and then work out how to apply to patients.

18

Self-Compassion

I have included self-compassion in this section as although it is not a key component of ACT per se, the integration of self-compassion-focused practice is able to mediate the ACT strategies that we have discussed and vice versa. Many therapists I know very much value and understand the role that self-compassion-focused practice can have when working with clients, particularly those in very complex emotional spaces such as when approaching the end of life. However, knowing how and when to engage in this practice can be difficult.

It is important to be aware of the implications of self-compassion practice within the end-of-life space. For many people that you are meeting with, they will be getting messages from the people around them (both within and outside of the health system) which will reinforce the ideas around being positive, and not allowing thoughts about difficult things to show up, and many patients will internalise these. In fact, many people will arrive at therapy naming the impact of feeling that they are not 'living up to' or 'feeling the ways that people seem to expect'. In this sense, a poorly placed discussion about self-compassion may run the risk of reinforcing these ideas that they are carrying around needing to be positive and optimistic (although this is clearly not the intention from a therapy perspective). In this context then, it is important to be clear about why the role of self-compassion is important, and the ways that they can apply it.

DOI: 10.4324/9781003431640-21

When speaking with patients about this, I will generally find myself introducing something like this:

> Wow, when you are speaking it is clear how much you are tuned into the other people in your world, and what their experience of this is. You seem to have huge amounts of compassion for their experiences and recognise how hard it is – but I wonder whether you are able to extend that same kindness to yourself?

Now, of course, this might look different depending on the context by which the conversation arises, but I have found that being explicit about the ways that the person is connecting with compassion to the people around them is a good gateway into exploring their own relationship to compassion, rather than the other way around, which may feel to them that it has come from no-where and be quite nebulous.

Self-compassion (and any discussion around gratitude) may be loaded for people who are approaching the end of life. It is likely that many people will be quite externally focused (usually with worry about what will happen to the people around them in the process of dying and post-death) which can mean that it will be harder for them to focus on the self-compassion work. In addition to this, you may find that they struggle to find language and words for how they would be able to be self-compassionate. If this is the case, using some of the strategies below will likely be useful. You may also encounter resistance to the idea of self-compassion, particularly when it is linked for the patient to the idea of how they show up in the face of their situation (for instance, if they perceive that to 'fight' the disease, they can't allow themselves to be compassionate).

Much of the self-compassion work will be reliant on you as the therapist recognising the cues by which to enact it. This is particularly true when the times that the compassion may be most helpful are those which are being driven by thoughts and emotions about how the person is showing up around their death, and can often be recognised by the 'shoulds' arriving in the therapy room. Most people will not recognise this in the compassion sphere, in the same way, that they would if they were not engaging in self care, or not sleeping properly for example, and as such you may find that the process of engaging them in discussions (and ultimately practice) around self-compassion may be something that needs to be revisited over and over.

The Compassionate Friend

This is a very well-known and well-used strategy in self compassion work but works very well in this population of people. As an extension of the introduction example explained above, the therapist is able to prompt people easily around using the analogy of being a compassionate friend. For example:

> Geez, I am just thinking here as you are speaking thinking, wowsers, this is so intense and hard for you. But it sounds like your brain is doing a great job of focusing on all of the things that you are missing rather than the things that you are doing well. I wonder what you would say to a friend in this situation?

Or

> I would imagine that if your friend was sitting here now, and I asked them how they think you are coping with all of this, they would say how well that you are doing given everything. They would recognise how tough it all is, and they would probably reach over and give you a hug to say 'mate, I can see how hard this is, and you are doing the best that you can'. I wonder what it would look like if you were able to be that kind to yourself?

Interestingly, in my experience, often these discussions will be filled with humour, and at times laughter. Although this sounds absurd in this context, many times people will be able to find their way to making sense of how hard that they are being on themselves, and recognise the 'self-deprecating voice' that shows up in this landscape. Within a safe therapy space, you can use this well to your advantage and explore the defences that arise for the person in the idea of recognising their own compassion.

'You are Doing the Best that You Can'

This sentence seems very simple, but can be incredibly powerful in working with self-compassion. Many people have not stopped to consider their role in their coping as they approach the end of life, as often they are caught within the physical and existential experience of trying to navigate everything that is happening – and so being explicit and naming this both can serve to highlight and model the ways in which they are coping, but also in bringing awareness to how they can be more self-compassionate.

I would often use this sentence in combination with doing some of the thinking about the character work that we have spoken about in the thought defusion chapter. Let's revisit our work with Susie.

Susie: I am not turning up for them – I am tired and exhausted at the end of the day, and when they arrive home from school, I want to be able to have the conversations, but I don't. And then I lay awake for most of the night thinking about how I am a terrible parent, and all that they are going to remember of me is that I was never there for them.

Therapist: Wow. That sounds really hard. Outside of what your brain is telling you, do you believe this is the case?

Susie: (Laughs uncomfortably) Yes. No. Sometimes. I mean, I don't want to believe it.

Therapist: And, and this is going to maybe be a hard question, but, what do you think the kids would say to that?

Susie: Now, they would agree. I am not able to do what they need from me.

Therapist: And, what about them in the future?

Susie: (Sobs) I don't know, I would hope that they would see it.

Therapist: (Pauses) I would imagine that they will. I wonder whether they would see the situation that you are in with a huge amount of compassion. (pauses). I am not sure if this will be helpful or not, but that's how I see where you are.

Susie: What do you mean?

Therapist: I see that in the face of such hardness, you are being intentional everyday to turn up to the kids every day, even when you are unwell, and when you don't have the energy for it. You are doing so much work for the future for them to make sure that they will be okay.

Susie: I guess so.

Therapist: But, your brain is getting stuck on the bits that it feels you aren't doing well enough. It's like that guy is showing up on your shoulder again, isn't it? That one that says that you aren't doing this well enough, or you aren't doing what you should be. But that guy is really predictable and familiar isn't he?

Susie: Yeah, he is always showing up.

Therapist: I wonder if there isn't another guy we could send in as well. I wonder if there is the guy who shows up to tell you that you are in a really tough spot, and even despite all the things that are hard, you are showing up the best way that you can?

Susie: (Pauses) Maybe.

Therapist: He probably won't be as loud as the not-doing-enough guy, but I wonder with paying more attention to the I'm-doing-the-best-I-can guy means that over time he might get louder.

When using this strategy, it is important to ensure that you do not get caught up in the content. Sometimes, as with this Susie, you may find that it would be easy to get into a push pull of all of the reasons that they are doing a great job, and that they are doing enough. That likely won't be very helpful, and will move the focus of the session from process to getting stuck in the content. Instead, using a concrete example above of how you have observed the patient behaving or showing up in the world, can be very powerful for a patient to hear, but you are not getting bogged down in trying to prove/disprove where they are.

19

Supporting People in Decision Making

At times people in these spaces will be faced with complex decisions. These decisions will usually be about starting or stopping a particular thing – and if it is about stopping, it will generally be a treatment that has some chance of making things better.

We often assume that there is a dichotomy about how people make sense of dying – with a sense of things either being in the 'treatment phase' or in the 'end-of-life phase'. The treatment phase will generally imply that there is something being done which may impact on the underlying disease process, such as chemotherapy, whereas the end-of-life phase may be seen as more focused on symptom management and trying to make someone's quality of life as good as possible for as long as possible.

And occasionally it is this straightforward – someone will recognise that the treatment that they have been having is not working, and is causing them too many side effects, and so they will opt to pursue what is often called 'best supportive care' or, closer to the end of life, might be called 'comfort measures'. This means, that there has been a decision made to not do anything to actively treat the underlying disease. I had a young patient in this situation just a couple of months ago, which when his cancer returned quickly after a surgery, and after several years of treatment (with his disease continuing to recur), he made the

DOI: 10.4324/9781003431640-22

choice to not have any more chemotherapy. He could recognise that in his decision the chemotherapy might give him a small survival benefit (measured in months likely) but that it would also come with significant side effects and other complications. And as such, he was comfortable in saying no to the option, instead choosing to focus on living the best that he could for as long as he could, with appropriate palliative care support.

However, for most people that we are seeing the decision is usually not as straightforward. For this young man, he had spent considerable time over the past years on treatment, and was very realistic and accepting of the situation that he was in. Even with a space of acceptance, many people will struggle to make an active choice to not engage in any treatment that may offer a space of hope.

We have spoken throughout the book about the role that hope and other complex emotions and how they show up – this space about decision making is a great example.

What is Driving This?

There are several pieces at play when we think about decision making at end of life. These include, but are definitely not limited to:

◆ *Everyone has a difference sense of reasonable risk.* I have met patients who will take on a potentially deadly treatment for the chance at 1% survival, and I have had others who will not do anything that compromises their quality of life at all. Most people will tend much more towards taking their chance with a treatment, even with the small chance that it may improve their overall situation. I have met haematology patients who have already had several unsuccessful bone marrow transplants who will decide to try another – whilst being able to clearly articulate that the risk of success (i.e. disease cure) would be less than 5%, whilst the risk of mortality and morbidity (dying from the procedure, of having significant changes to the *quality* of life) would be in the order of 90%. They would normally say to me something like 'Well if I don't have it, my chance of death is 100%. That is better than the 60% chance of dying from the process'. Every person who reads this will likely have a different idea about whether that is reasonable or not, but it is not an uncommon thing to come up in your clinical practice.

◆ *It may not be simple medically.* We assume that there will be a direct relationship between treatment and death, but for many complex diseases this is not the case. Within an oncology setting for instance, people will have chemotherapy to manage pain and slow disease spread, even if it is very clear it will not change the overall trajectory of the disease it will usually ensure an improved quality of life (somewhat paradoxical I know!).

◆ *It's harder to say no, than to just keep going.* When a person makes a decision to stop treatment it is much harder in many ways than just keeping on. If you think about the landscape in which people will make decisions about treatment, they are usually not making them in isolation – they have families and partners and friends who all have ideas and thoughts about what they should do. It is rare that someone would be able to stop treatment and have everyone in their world to be supportive of it. This happens often in the work that I do with young people, where the young people themselves will tell me that they have had enough and don't want to keep going, but continue to do so (even when the side effects are bad, and it feels futile) because it would be devastating to their families to consider that they had 'given up'.

◆ *Stopping is loaded.* Continuing on from the above, there is usually a dichotomy of the language and process around illness – you are either 'battling it' or you have 'lost the fight (these might seem extreme, but I would hear these words being used in this way many times a week). People will often fail to recognise even for themselves, that they are not doing either of these things by prioritising what feels best for them.

◆ *Hope and survival instinct are very strong.* That young man that I described is the exception. It is incredibly hard for people to make the decision to lean into the process awaiting them around death and dying. I don't mean that in the sense that they want to accelerate the process or anything like it, but by removing the option of treatment, it requires that someone then processes the fixed outcome of death, in a way that they have might not before. Hope particularly will drive most of the decision making around this – I have had patients who are suffering incredibly from treatments and not able to do any of the things that they have identified as important, in the knowledge that not only is their treatment not working, but that the cost of that treatment is very significant – but they will clearly state, this is my 'only hope' and 'I will take the chance, even if it is very small'.

◆ *Often the medical/treating teams will encourage the hope.* This is particularly true in younger patients, but it may be that the teams will also connect with the idea that they might be the exception and this treatment might be the one that turns things around. When patients say no to something, that also presents a challenge for teams. Thinking about the young man above, it was evident in our team that we all bumped into a sense of feeling helpless and impotent, even though he was in very good hands with the palliative care team.

◆ *There is no 100% right answer.* Even for experienced clinicians it can be difficult to accurately prognosticate about the time that someone has left, and this is even more complex when stopping treatment. There is no certainty that stopping the treatment will accelerate the disease process, nor is there any guarantee that staying on the treatment will reduce the speed. It can be incredibly hard for patients to navigate these decisions knowing that it is unlikely they will ever find a space of knowing and accepting 100% that they have made the right decision.

How to Navigate These Conversations

It goes without saying that these are delicate conversations. If someone is arriving in therapy wanting to talk about these things, there is a reasonable chance that they have not made a decision about what they want to do, and are seeking support in decision making. Some people may have an agenda of asking you for direct guidance, but this is not normally the case. People will use the therapy space to put language to the thoughts they are having but be unable to share anywhere else (particularly with friends and family who have their own vested interest in them continuing with treatment). They may not have thought about the consequences of stopping treatment in any real way – instead, they may have focused on the immediacy of relief of stopping the side effects but may not have thought through the next steps of what would happen with their disease and approach to end of life.

I remember a young man with leukaemia who wanted to stop treatment – he had advanced disease and was approaching end of life – the treatment that he was having was keeping the disease somewhat at bay, but he was continuing to deteriorate. When I asked him what he thought would happen when he stopped treatment his answer surprised me. This was someone who had many brushes with death since his diagnosis and he could tell me how bad his disease was, but, when he thought about stopping treatment, he had pictured that he would go home, go back to school and carry on.

We have spoken many times throughout the book about the idea of the escape fantasy, and treatment decision making can be a great example of it. As above, the brain tries to help the person in giving them lots of thoughts about how hard it is on treatment, and how it is to manage the effects of it, but then sometimes won't identify the bits that come after the escape fantasy (a little like wanting to hasten death, as we spoke about way back in Chapter 4).

In exploring these conversations with people, it is really important to get a sense of what their understanding is, and as an extension of that, an understanding of how they are framing the steps around what it would mean to stop something.

It can be particularly important to be explicit about naming the complexity of this decision, and that even though thinking about the next steps is hard it is important to talk through these so that they are able to be aware and connect with the decisions that they are making.

An example conversation might look like:

Client: I have just had enough. I can't do it anymore. I have spent since last treatment in hospital with fever and pain, and what's worse, the scans I had last week said that the spots have stayed pretty much the same.

Therapist: That must have been really disappointing – I know that we have spoken before about how hopeful you were that this might be the drug that would make the big changes.

Client: Yeah, I was. And I am due for it again tomorrow, but I am thinking now that I don't want to bother with it all.

Therapist: You mean stopping?

Client: Yeah, is that bad?

Therapist: Bad? I don't think it's a bad decision, but I think it's a decision that you probably need to think through pretty carefully. How is it sitting with you at the moment?

Client: I am struggling. On the one hand, it's terrible. The treatment, I can't imagine living the rest of my life like this. But then again, if I don't do the treatment, I won't have much of a life, so maybe it's an easy decision.

Therapist: Have you spoken to your doctor about it?

Client: No. I don't want her to think that I am giving up. She isn't giving up on me.

Therapist: Is that what it would feel like if you didn't keep going with treatment? Giving up?

Client: Well, I would die. They told me that I don't have any other options, and if this drug is keeping it stable, then the risk is that when I stop, it will just take off. That's what it was doing before I started this.

Therapist: It's hard, isn't it? Because my guess is that there is no right answer to such a big decision.

Client: What do you mean? If it means that I am going to die, then it is almost not a decision.

Therapist: Well, as you have been talking it has struck me that there isn't much that is a 100% known in all of this. Right now, we know that the tumours are stable on the drug, but that being on that drug is making you miserable and getting in the way of you living the way you want to be. But we don't know what happens next – the drug could keep working, or it might stop working, or you could stop the drug and the cancer might take off, or it might stay in hibernation for a while.

Client: That's true. I would hope that I would stop it, and they would just stay there and not change, I could manage that.

Therapist: I am not sure how you might get the answer for that. I think instead of trying to manage all of the potential options for what might happen, there might be more to do around being intentional about your decision making about this – that's the only bit you can really control. So, what are your options in that?

Client: Well, I stop the drug, or I continue it.

Therapist: That's true. Are there any others?

Client: I don't think so.

Therapist: Well, I guess we haven't explored what your options might be in continuing on the drug – your doctor might have some other meds that help manage the side effects, or spacing out your cycles like you have done before.

Client: That's true – I haven't thought about those.

Therapist: It sounds like you need to have a conversation with your doctor about it, and really understand what the options are so that you can make a decision that is based on some more information.

Client: Do you have other patients do this? Give up on it all because it is too hard?

Therapist: It's an interesting question – it's a conversation that I have with people all the time. But, it can be really tough to stop treatment. Most people think about it, though. Is that how you are thinking about it? You have mentioned giving up a couple of times now. What does that mean to you?

Client: (Pauses) Yeah, I think so. Well, if I stop, I am going to die. So that's giving up, isn't it?

Therapist: Mmm. I don't know. I think that for many people I see, they would say that they have to think about what life they are living on treatment versus having a limited time. As we have talked about before, you have made sense of knowing that you have a limited time, and so it makes sense to me that you would be thinking about how you want to be spending that time – and if that time comes at the cost of being really unwell, I think most people would be thinking about what it would look like to try and make things feel better, even for a shorter time.

Client: But, what if I stop and the treatment is doing something? I will have thrown away that chance.

Therapist: I think this is the piece that is important to make sure that you have all of the information that you can to help you in this. This is a huge decision to make, and there is the piece about having the information that you need, but the other piece is about being sure that you are committed to it. We have talked lots about escape fantasy, do you think some of this is coming into play now?

Client: Maybe. I can recognise that I want to run away from the treatment because it is hard, but then when I really think about it, I am terrified of what happens next.

Therapist: I wonder whether this is one of those situations where being present might be helpful. Right here and right now, it sounds like your intention is to show up for treatment tomorrow – is that correct?

Client: Yes, I think so.

Therapist: And we recognise that there is a bunch of stuff going on which might mean that this changes in the future – but for now, if you are planning on turning up, I wonder how we might recognise the intentionality in this.

Client: What do you mean?

Therapist: Well, it sounds like part of what is showing up in all of this is lots of chatter in your mind about what it would be like to stop, and how that would be different, but you are not ready to do that right now. So, I wonder what would look different in your mind if instead of focusing on how you might escape it, you leaned into the decision. What would happen to that chatter if you told yourself 'I am making the decision to show up for treatment today – even though it is hard'.

Client: I don't know. It would probably feel that I am less trapped by it.

Therapist: It's funny, isn't it? My patients will often say to me that they have no choice about things, or that they feel trapped. But, you could say right now, I am not going to have any more treatment. But right now, you are choosing to keep on with it.

When discussing the decision making process it can be easy to get caught up in content – this is the exact thing that we should try and avoid in therapy (both from an ACT perspective, but also in recognising that this is likely going to mirror how everyone else is showing up for them in this). You will notice in the example above, that in these conversations you may span across many aspects of the hexaflex, but also circle back to ACT strategies and ways of conceptualising things that have come up for them in the past. It would be unlikely that the first conversation that you have with someone will be about decision making, and so, when this arises it is important to help people to recognise all of the skills, they have to navigate this, but also in their capacity to show up to difficult and hard things.

If they did make the decision to stop treatment, it is likely that there will be fallout for them – even in those patients where people will tell them it is 'their choice' or that they 'will support them in whatever they do', the people around them will likely have some response to this, and so in the conversation with your patients it can be helpful to anticipate this with them and explore how they might address it. Usually, simple prompt questions will open the discussion easily (most of what drives complex decision making is the awareness of how others will respond, and so the patients will likely engage easily in this process).

An example might be:

'It is a big decision to change what you are doing here – how do you think your people will make sense of it?'

Or

'Do you have any worries about how the people in your world will respond to this?'

When working in the space of decision making it is important to recognise that there can be an oscillation and changing space for the people that you see – it may be that they discuss frequently the ideas of stopping treatment, or changing their options, but may not take any action towards this. As therapists it is important for us to recognise the utility for people in this process – it may be for a sense of control, it may be connecting with a passive suicidal ideation, or it may have another origin. Sometimes, the person that you are speaking with will not be able to recognise the utility of this process, and may require some engagement with yourself around connecting with the underlying reasons that they are struggling with the decision making. Just like many other things we have discussed so far, the therapist brings their own ideas/biases/projections about what they think the patient should do or not do. It is important to explore these in supervision, but also in thinking about how these show up in your interactions with the patient.

Part 3

The Therapist Process

It would be remiss to not include a section in the book about the impact that doing this work has on therapists. It is universally recognised that there is a 'cost' of being a therapist, however, we equally know that doing this work, particularly in the context of end of life is very satisfying and deeply engaging. A good measure of this in the absence of others is that of staff turnover, with anecdotally many services experiencing almost no turnover in their therapy teams, and the experience of having people stay within roles for decades being commonplace.

There have been volumes of work done exploring the ways that the ideas and experience of the therapeutic process impact those who are involved – both from the perspective of the client and of the therapist. However, in the work of palliative care, this has been less well examined. Most of the work in this space has focused on the role of burnout and making sense of the cost of compassion, and turning up consistently in the face of the suffering of others. Furthermore, the work has been focused on those who are involved in direct care – nurses and doctors working in hospitals, hospices and community settings delivering hands-on care to those who are end of life, rather than those who are working directly with the emotional experience of patients and their families.

The following section is intentionally meant to be self-reflective. You may or not may not recognise many of the aspects that are discussed, however, it is important to pause and

DOI: 10.4324/9781003431640-23

explore why this is the case. As part of training, most therapists are exposed to ideas of strict boundaries and tight emotional regulation around connection with their patients – however, working with those who are approaching the end of life means that these boundaries by necessity look different, or you may find that relationships that are held therapeutically will also be held differently by the therapist.

When working with many supervisees they will talk about the idea of the shifting expectations in this space. For most people when they come into this work, they will hold worry or anxiety about not knowing what to do (or even a fear of coping with the death work), however, most people early on, recognise that it is not the death that is the hardest part. Most people will find that it is the spaces in between – the waiting for something to happen, the knowledge of things going poorly but not being sure how badly, and the waiting to die. These are the spaces that therapists provide, hold and often feel ineffectual in. This isn't a reflection on clinical skill – it is simply a reflection of the difficulty of the space.

Bumping into the bigness of death, and all of the pieces around it is definitely not something to be underestimated. Nor, is the cost on the human who sits in the face of it and walks alongside their patients, many of which they will feel quite connected to. As therapists, there is often a parallel process that occurs with our patients – when things are going well we, too, connect with this, and the same occurs when your patients are feeling stuck, overwhelmed, or deeply saddened.

20

What Shows Up for Us

There is a significant cost to the people who sit in the spaces of the unknown. This has been demonstrated over and over in various studies and settings, and palliative care and end-of-life work are no exception. There are high rates of compassion fatigue and burnout in those who work in this space, and this is often exacerbated in situations where clinicians will identify a sense of powerlessness or having to work outside of their values.

To work in a therapeutic capacity not only are therapists recognising and being present to the unfixable nature – we are leaning into it, and connecting to the pieces around it. We will need to sit with discomfort (both our own and our patients') and we will likely be confronted by our own ideas of death and dying. One of the most challenging ideas that can arise in this space is around the concept of a good death – each of us will bring different ideas and measures of what a good death looks like, and by extension how we would define a 'bad death'.

This of course is only one side of the coin – and it would be unreasonable to only focus on the ways in which this costs us. Many people who work in this space connect readily with the things that the work gives – a connection with what is truly important, relationships and engagement in the moments that really matter and the opportunity to do very meaningful work

DOI: 10.4324/9781003431640-24

that transcends the session itself, with flow on into the patients' people and their people.

Working primarily in the Adolescent and Young Adult (AYA) cancer space for the last 15 years, my role has meant that I have had very significant relationships with patients develop, and I have been with many of these same young people when they have been approaching the end of their lives. It is in these conversations that I have experienced the power of being in the moment with another human trying to make sense of the completely unimaginable. It is in these same moments that I have shared connection and laughter and genuine grief. Many of these conversations are still in my brain, mostly in the form of a snapshot in time, but some of them have disappeared.

In order to do this work, we need to be open to understanding a) the impact on us (good or bad) and b) the way that we show up to it (both for our patients and for ourselves).

Early in our careers, we are more likely to be disparaging of the emotions and feelings that arise – fearful that allowing them in may mean that we are not able to have 'boundaries' the way that we should. But, later on, as I have noticed in my own practice small moments of reflection may allow you to understand the ways that you are making space for these challenges and how you show up to them.

When working in this space, it is easy to feel a sense of normality – about emotion, and the ways in which humans suffer and the experiences of being close to death. But, it is important to take time to synthesise how strange this work is! In your personal life, across your lifespan you may have exposure to a handful of people that you are connected to, but in this work, we build strong intimate connections with hundreds if not thousands of people, and if you are working primarily with people at the end of life, you will be exposed to the cumulative grief around that same space.

Therefore, in order to be able to do the work, you need to work out how you can manage the stuff that comes with it.

Some of the main things that may show up for people in this space are:

◆ *Being more aware of emotions in session/out of session.* The conversations that happen in this space require us to focus not only on the client experience, but also on our own thoughts and cognitions about this. Depending on what is happening in our lives the content of sessions and interactions may permeate in a different way that you might have experienced before.

◆ *It is unpredictable.* Most people assume when starting this work that it will be the death and dying stuff that presents the biggest challenge for clinicians, and sometimes it is, but just as often the most distressing situations will come from a sense of therapeutic impotence, or of not knowing what to do next. It may come from a conversation, or a moment of acknowledgement in a session. It is important to recognise these things when they happen, there will likely be a pattern even though it will feel like it comes from nowhere every single time.

◆ *You will bump into your own death stuff.* This is unavoidable, and pretty challenging. But it isn't necessarily a bad thing, but it will make you think about your own mortality in a way that you haven't before – it may also make you think about how you want to be showing up to life. (If I think about the ways that this has shown up in the people I supervise, it invariably causes some interesting reflections and connections with the ways that they spend their time).

◆ *You may be convinced that you will die at any time.* No bones about it, being surrounded by death all the time will make you assume that you, too, will experience some random diagnosis that will lead to you being in the same situation as one of your patients. This is particularly true when the patient shares similar characteristics to you (kids the same age, grew up in the same place, being in the same life stage). Usually, this means that people will become much more hypervigilant about their health, and at the extreme end become quite anxious about what might happen to them.

The next couple of chapters will speak about the ways that this might show up, how you might recognise the impact on yourself, and what to do with it.

21

Managing Our Own Stuff

As we move through the world as humans, but also as therapists we become collectors. We collect ideas, stories, feelings, identities, cognitive pathways, and interpersonal skills (plus a bunch of other stuff). It is well established in psychotherapy practice that in order to be a good therapist, you also need to identify and recognise your own stuff and how it shows up for you. This is of course multidirectional and changeable – the client relationships that were challenging at one stage of your career might look different now, and as we move through our own lives, we also change the way that we process and make sense of things.

I was reflecting on this a couple of days ago when I was writing a condolence card to the family of one of my young patients. I have done this routinely since I began working in this space, but as I sat down and wrote the words done, I was able to recognise the change. In the past, I would have written something that felt safer – 'I was so sorry to hear about _____. I am sure that in this difficult time you are all finding ways to support each other, but if you need anything, please reach out'.

The note I wrote a couple of days ago looked somewhat different – 'I was so sad to hear about _____. I feel incredibly lucky to have been able to spend time with her, and to share in the way that she made sense of such a tricky world. It was always a pleasure to work with her, and with all of you. You are all in my thoughts'.

DOI: 10.4324/9781003431640-25

You may say that these things aren't that different – and in some ways they aren't, but I feel different in my thinking about them – that relationship was very important to me, we had gotten to know each other over many years, and we had walked alongside her family as they navigated the brutality of being a young person dying of cancer. There wasn't a time that she didn't smile when I entered the room. That smile will stay with me.

Therapists are usually drawn to therapy for a particular reason – and that reason is usually rooted somewhere in our early life experiences. I am not necessarily encouraging you to go deep diving in this, but I would encourage you to think a little bit about what your experiences of death, grief and processing the things around your family dynamics (we all have them, let's face it!) are, so that when you bump into situations that either mirror them, or conversely, presenting in an unfamiliar way, you are able to recognise what might be at play. It seems that as we as therapists develop over time, these things become more obvious and noticeable to us when they show up, but if you are relatively new in your career you might not yet have stumbled across it.

There are a couple of things to consider when we think about managing our own stuff in this space:

◆ *It's harder to maintain boundaries.* I don't mean that this is permission to have flagrant boundary violations, but the nature of the patients that we will see at end of life will therapeutically look quite different. When we work in disciplines where patients are complex in regards to their mental health or behaviours, we are much more likely to be cognisant of keeping very tight boundaries – but when working with people at end of life, they are often people who have been without pathology or significant pre-existing concerns and will want to see us about things that we can relate to. This means that we need to be even more cognisant of how we show up in these relationships.

◆ *We are humans first, therapists second.* Much of what happens therapeutically when working with people at the end of life is about relationship and connection more than techniques or strategies. It is the moments of being present in the unfixable and the recognition of limited time that makes this work so meaningful, but of course, the flipside is that we are likely to bump into more complexity of emotion in this space. What is happening to our patients is also going to happen to us, and that can be very difficult for us to get our heads around.

◆ *Being human also means emotions will show up*. Part of learning to be a therapist is learning to keep your emotions in check – we do lots of work around boundaries, and transference issues, but we often don't take the time (or the self-compassion) to allow us to experience genuine grief and sadness when it arises. The reality of this work is that you will have deep and intimate connections with people, and those people will die. It is important to recognise and manage how this shows up for you – lots of people expect sadness, but may instead feel a sense of relief, or conversely, they may find that they are angry with the circums-tances of someone's death. All of this is of course fine, but you need to work out how to manage this in a productive way (and to keep it contained from your clinical work). It is good to get into the practice of being cognisant of the presence of these emotions and using supervision to understand the function and process around managing them.

If you have read these paragraphs and felt quite worried – don't be. The highest level of anxiety for new therapists working in this space is often about not knowing how they will react when difficult things show up, and many people are fearful of not knowing what to say (or saying the wrong thing) in these really important discussions. The work that you will do at the end of life is of course very important, but it can be helpful to recognise that much of what you will do in this space is based on the same skills that you have developed across your practice:

1. *Slow down* – Even in the face of wanting to speed up, intentionally slow down. We make mistakes when we try and move too quickly.
2. *Show up and be present* – Tune into what the person in front of you is telling you, and notice what is happening for them in that moment.
3. *Be curious* – get to know the process of how it is for them, connect with where they are and understand what they need (from therapy, from you, and in general).
4. *Be quiet* – allowing space in these conversations will facilitate more. Don't be tempted to fill the space. This is particularly important after an 'I don't know' – if you wait, the answer will come.
5. *Resist strategies* – In a space of uncertainty, or feeling that things are unfixable the thing that we will usually call on is a raft of strategies. When you notice that this is happening (it is often accompanied by a sense of 'spinning' and not knowing what to do next) go back to step one.
6. *Recognise that you are human* – not every session will be brilliant, and some will feel terrible. Our ability to assess this isn't great, though, and you have no way of knowing what the person has taken away.
7. *Be kind* – We are able to do this easily to our clients, but it wouldn't hurt to extend this to yourself as well.

22

Tolerance of Sitting

Within ACT frameworks and throughout this book, we have spoken about the idea of sitting with discomfort and holding spaces. We all know that to be a 'good therapist' we have to allow the person sitting in front of us to have space – and being in that space means that there isn't much room designated for us – that is the role, and that is how we can do the work we do.

But, when working with end of life, the 'stuff' that occupies the space that we are holding is challenging, and simply sitting with it may present a sense of impotence and discomfort that even experienced therapists are not familiar with.

I had a conversation with one of my supervisees over the past couple of weeks. She had been presented with a tricky situation – a long-term patient of hers that she was quite fond of, had found out that her disease had become incurable, and was, of course, distressed by this. Session after session, the patient had arrived with acute and unsettled emotion – filling the walls with loud sobs, and expressing the unmentionable distress of having to reconcile the idea of leaving her children when they weren't old enough to remember her. The supervisee had left all of these sessions feeling completely helpless – she could recognise her own sense of having nothing to add, and largely unknowing of what to say. She knew intellectually that she wouldn't be able to offer anything that would alleviate the woman's suffering – and yet, when that relief didn't arise, she

DOI: 10.4324/9781003431640-26

was shocked and found herself reflecting on her own therapeutic competence.

> I know that other people would have known what to do,
> but I couldn't think of anything. I bet you would have
> known what to say. What would you have said?

This is a familiar space when working at the end of life, but generally of therapy. In the cloistered walls of the therapy room there
are no check points – all we have to guide us about 'success' is the
outward signs and communication of the person in front of us.
Sometimes, with experience, we can judge well that things have
gone well, or poorly, but these are usually at the extreme ends –
the subtle nuance of the sessions in between are much more open
to interpretation (or more accurately misinterpretation).

In all of this, and the chatter that happens in our minds –
about what we should be doing, and what the patient needs,
and how we could be better therapists – we find ourselves
forgetting the really important bit.

Most of the time, there is nothing to be said.

Sitting in a room, silent and in the presence of intense
emotion is an unquestionably hard thing to do. We can safely
anticipate that for therapists a couple of things will happen:

◆ *We will acknowledge the space* – and we will understand
  the importance of the space. We can recognise that for
  many people we see, that therapeutic space may be the
  only space that they will ever have to explore such
  difficult concepts and emotions.
◆ *Our brains will spin* – Even if we see and recognise the
  need to sit, our brain is likely to kick in and come up
  with a million strategies and ideas that we can offer the
  person to 'help' them work through it. This process is
  much more about us than the patient, and if we catch the
  spinning it will allow us to sit and hold those thoughts
  within ourselves.
◆ *Difficult stuff will come up for us* – difficult thoughts and
  emotions likely. The thoughts may be around the things

that we could do, or not do or the experience of the person. The emotion that may arise will likely be intense and be a little bit about the patient, but much more about us – we might be observing the sadness in them and feeling this acutely. This is really important to acknowledge – most people will be pretty uncomfortable about this, but it is part of being in a therapeutic interaction where you care for the other person. Holding that emotion is fine, expressing that emotion to your patient and requiring their support is not. If this is happening, this is the kind of thing to take to supervision.

◆ *In silence, there will likely be progress.* Noticing our brains telling us to jump in and try and give a solution is a great prompt to remind us to slow down and lean into the space, even if it is uncomfortable. Some of the best interventions and therapy sessions will come from letting the difficult stuff hang in the air, with the patient bringing all of the threads together.

23

Saying Goodbye

In so many ways, it is hard to do this chapter justice. To try and condense down the ways that we process the grief and sadness about a patient dying within a couple of thousand words seems inadequate somehow, but in many ways, it could be said with much less.

> The reality of working with people at the end of life is that many of those people (not necessarily all) will die, and more than likely you will be sad about some of them (again, not necessarily all). And that is okay (and isn't about breaking boundaries).

We have talked throughout the book about the ways in which this work challenges the ways that we might think about boundaries, and the ways that they show up, and so I won't revisit this here, but it is very likely that these will show up around having to say goodbye to patients. Sometimes you may find yourself knowing that a patient has a very short time left, or you may recognise that it is your last session before they become too unwell to engage with you. Alternatively, you may not get the opportunity to recognise this before a patient dies, and you are left with navigating the emotions around this.

Either way, it is important to think about what is for you, and what is for the patient.

DOI: 10.4324/9781003431640-27

For example, I know of many clinicians who will go and see patients when the strict therapeutic work might be done. This can be because the patient wants them to keep coming – this is really common in those patients for whom you have had a regular or long-term relationship, and they will likely see you as a person who comes, versus the therapist per se (this is particularly true in working with young people, where you may have had a long-term relationship, or a pattern of seeing them whenever they are in hospital – changing that relationship at the end is likely to be distressing to them even if you don't feel that you are doing therapeutic things anymore!)

For navigating this, let the patient and family be the guide – for some they will want you to keep coming, others will not have the tolerance. They will tell you, and sometimes it can be helpful to leave it with them, for example – 'I know that everything is taking lots of energy for you at the moment, and I don't want to take that energy away from other things, but very happy to see you if it is helpful – I will leave it with you to reach out if you want to catch up?' Most of the time, at this stage of life, people won't reach out.

Of, course there is the other side of that coin, is that you are doing it for you.

You are sad that someone is dying, and you go to see them for that 'one last time'. Although on the surface this sounds like it would be completely inappropriate, but in many ways, it can help us make sense of what is going on, and as such, can be very helpful (I will caveat this with the idea of limit, duration and patient needs being very important in this – if the family or the patient don't want you to go, under no circumstances do you do that! Also, saying goodbye once is okay, doing it everyday is not). If you are doing this, you need to be clear for yourself about why you are doing it, and what this facilitates for you. For me personally, I find it helpful to make sense of the death itself – I have known countless people who have died, and seeing them in the final stages allows my brain to make sense of knowing that they are not going to recover. I also find that the families have incredible comfort from having a familiar face come to see them (particularly if the care team has changed from the main treating team to palliative or supportive care, where the re-lationships might be newer and less established).

The actual saying goodbye is a really personal thing – I don't think I have ever verbalised a goodbye to a patient, I will just be present in knowing that it is the last time. There will sometimes be mutual collusion with the patient, where you both know it is the end, but the pretence of catching up again is held.

And sometimes, the patient will say a simple thank you. Even though it will be tempting to respond or to defuse this (as it usually will make therapists feel pretty uncomfortable), notice it, and accept it humbly. You don't know what difference you have made to someone, and it is important to them for you to know.

When a patient dies you may have a couple of responses –

◆ *You could feel lots of things* – this might be when you have a patient that you are particularly close to, or if things haven't gone well with the death (or the way that they or you were hoping for), or it might be the first time that you are bumping into death in this way. If this happens, notice what is going on for you, and take the time that you need, come up with some rituals that feel helpful, and chat with your supervisor/colleagues about how they manage this stuff. Sometimes, this will catch us off guard – it might be a patient you weren't particularly connected to, or it may intersect with something in your life. Either way, the main thing is to be kind to yourself in all of this.

◆ *You might not feel much at all* – this is also okay. Sometimes we connect less with some patients than others, or the death might be expected and feel okay. It may be that you have had a bunch of people die all at once, and you didn't connect with all of them in the same way. If this happens occasionally, it is probably nothing to worry about, but if you find yourself being more and more disconnected from the thoughts around death, or not connecting with the emotions around it, it is important to explore why (and check in around burnout – people doing this work are at very high risk).

It is a personal choice often about going to the funerals of patients. Therapists are in a strange place with this – if you don't know whether the person has disclosed that they are going to therapy, you may well be in a strange position if someone were to ask who you are! Also, although it is commonplace for nurses and doctors to attend funerals for some patients, they would rarely attend all – and so, if you are going to go, you need to think about why – is it for you, is it for the family, is it appropriate? Sometimes, we can do our own rituals and process around making sense of this, without having to attend a funeral.

In our team, we rarely go to funerals. In fact, now I would only go if the family specifically asked me to. Personally, I find that attending them makes the grief harder for me, as I am then faced with them as a person outside of the time that I knew them. I see pictures of them with their friends, and get a sense of them before their disease – which for me makes it much harder to make sense of the loss. This is just my experience, and others may experience it very differently.

We have spoken throughout the book about the cost that this work can have, but it isn't all cost – to work with people at this stage of their lives is beautiful and powerful work to do, and allows us to also be present to what is important in our own worlds. Remembering the work and the connection can be a powerful buffer to the cost of the death itself.

Part 4

Clinical Case Studies

The purpose of this section isn't to give you scripts or answers about how to approach particular issues or problems, however, they are meant to act as prompts to develop thinking about some of the ways that ACT can be applied. Some of these responses may be familiar to other sections of the book, but applied in a different context, or in a different way. These are short little snippets of conversation and a little bit by way of introduction to the person. It isn't unusual in end of life work that you may get incomplete or time-critical referrals, and it may not be until you are in the room that you have any real sense of what the presenting concern is. I would encourage you in approaching these to think about how you would approach a particular scenario, or how you might respond. We often do our best learning in an experiential way, and so thinking about how you would tailor the conversation to your own style, or to progress your own strategies/interventions will be helpful.

I would encourage you to show up to these cases with a sense of curiosity, not only for what is going on for the person you are reading about but also for yourself as the therapist.

It will also be helpful (although sometimes much harder) to identify the ways in which the presentations might result in you feeling stuck, unsure or even incompetent. Working through a case study will absolutely not stop this showing up in the clinical room, but noticing your own experience and what you

DOI: 10.4324/9781003431640-28

are bringing cognitively to the case is a helpful directional marker of what to do, but conversely, what not to do.

Within psychotherapy, there is an adage around the idea of doing the opposite of what you feel that you should be doing, which arose out of the work of Melanie Klein. Now, of course, ACT and child psychoanalysis are quite different, but within the End of life context, it is very common to feel the urge to jump in and do something – when the best thing you can do is to sit with your own discomfort and not do anything at all, and await the patient to respond/elaborate/continue. You will notice through these cases, there is considerable mention of the pauses and the spaces in therapy – don't underestimate these, this is often where the best work is done.

It is important to note (as has been the case all through the book) that these case studies are composites of many people with similar presenting concerns, if they appear familiar it is a coincidence, but may be reflective that you have encountered or navigated similar presentations before. You may also be shocked at the directness of some of the conversations about death and suffering – this is a reflection of what we have mentioned earlier in the book – many people who are seeking therapy at the end of life are very open about discussing the crux of what is going on, with the energy for euphemism feeling less present. Conversely, you will notice that for a couple of these examples, the conversations are much less overt. Both of these are fine, it's about noticing how you, the patient and the dynamic are showing up in the room on the day.

24

Managing Physical Decline

The experience of physical decline is something that is likely to happen to all people at the end of life. Sometimes this occurs in a metered and gradual way or conversely, it may be fast and brutal. In both instances, most people will find it difficult to make adjustments to the ways that their bodies are working/ not working and often will hold a sense of betrayal around the same.

Thomas is a 50 year old who has recently been diagnosed with metastatic lung cancer. He suspects that he got it from working on construction sites when he was younger, but his doctor has told him they aren't able to confirm this. Prior to his diagnosis he was working as a manager on a commercial building site, but had noticed getting breathless walking up and down the stairs at work. His wife had suggested he go to the GP, and was then completely shocked and surprised by the diagnosis, and within weeks of investigation, he was started on treatment. His disease was shown to be in his bones and brain, as well as his lungs. In the past months, he has noticed a decline in his physical functioning, and he is struggling more and more to complete the tasks that he was able to do just prior to diagnosis.

Thomas: It's like I am useless – I can't even help Marilyn with the shopping anymore. That was always my job. I would go to the shops on a Friday afternoon and pick up what we needed. She doesn't even ask me to

DOI: 10.4324/9781003431640-29

do it anymore – she can see what it does to me, and how angry I get when it happens.

Therapist: What do you think that anger is about?

Thomas: Frustration mostly, I think. I just want to be able to do the things that I could always do. Now I am stuck in this useless body, and it is getting worse day by day.

Therapist: You are noticing the changes that often?

Thomas: It's impossible not to. Maybe not each day, but week to week. And the terrifying thing is, I know that it isn't getting any better. And it can't get better. This is it for me now.

Therapist: Wow. That is a lot to process. (Pauses) What is your brain doing with that?

Thomas: What can I do? It just what it is. I am now that guy who is useless and a waste of space.

Therapist: Can I check something with you? It feels to me, and tell me if I am wrong, but it sounds like there are two parts of you turning up in this? The one part is the bit that is angry and frustrated and struggling to know what to do with all of this, and then there is another part that jumps in and says 'It is what it is'. It sounds like that voice is shutting down the other parts, the parts that are maybe harder to experience if you connect with them.

Thomas: Well, there isn't much point in thinking about it if I am going to die anyway. What is the point of torturing myself, or for that matter everyone around me?

Therapist: So, does it feel easier to stay disconnected from it?

Thomas: Maybe. (Pauses for some time) Except, that I am not, not really. It is in my face every day. Look at my legs, I can't even walk in here by myself anymore. And this pain.

Therapist: This might sound like a strange question, but what is the cost of staying disconnected from it? Particularly when it sounds like it is showing up regardless?

Thomas: I don't know. I think it is just the irritability. I try not to connect with it, and keep my brain away, and then I notice something that I can't do, and when everything feels hard, it makes me realise. And then, that's when the frustration really shows up.

Therapist: So, I wonder if you gave it space, perhaps that might change how it shows up. But it isn't simple, right? There is a benefit to keeping it shut down as well?

Thomas: (Pauses, and becomes teary) Sometimes, I can have some minutes where I don't think about it, and then I feel normal for a second.

Therapist: (Sits silently for some time and then speaks gently) You know how we have talked before about naming things, I wonder what happens if we name all of the stuff that is showing up here as grief?

Thomas: What would that do? How would it change anything? It's not going to stop it.

Therapist: I am not sure (pauses) but this stuff is showing up for a reason. As you speak, and watching how things are changing for you over the time that we have spent together, I can see the weight that all of this is. I wonder whether naming it might not shift it, but it may allow you to see it in a different way?

Thomas: Maybe. (Sits silently)

Therapist: Can we explore the elephant in the room?

Thomas: Oh yeah. You are always wanting to bring that bloody elephant in! (Laughs)

Therapist: I think we need to talk about the comment that you made before, that you are noticing the change happening every day, in your body. I can't help thinking that your brain is working really hard not to think about what that means, but it is showing up anyway.

Thomas: Yeah. (Becomes teary)

Therapist: And, from the outside looking in, that fight looks really exhausting. And, is probably getting in the way of things.

Thomas: Yeah. (Sits silently). Yeah, it is. It's in my mind all the time – how the best of my days have already passed, and now it is only going to get worse. And I see it.

I can't stop thinking about it. (Pauses) But there isn't any point dwelling on it is there? It is just what it is.

Therapist: I am not sure if you caught it, but I think your brain has just jumped back into the space of shutting down the other parts.

Thomas: Yeah.

Therapist: I think it's important that we pause and connect here – like lots of the other things that we have talked about, it may not be helpful to go there – you are the expert in this, and so if it feels too hard, or not the right time, that's okay. I do wonder though, whether even just noticing that it has happened might be helpful. It seems to me that when that happens, it is your brain jumping in to say, 'Woah, it's too hard/too much/too painful right now, so back off' and that's not good or bad, but it might be worth noticing particularly if the other tricky stuff shows up around it, like the irritability or frustration.

Case Study Reflections:

1. In Thomas' case, what were the things that jumped out at you before you read the transcript?
2. What ACT-congruent frameworks/interventions do you notice in the discussion?
3. What are any different moves/directions would you have taken to the therapist?
4. When, if ever, did you feel stuck? If you think about this patient presenting to you, are there any spaces where you might feel stuck, or unsure where to go?
5. Where would you go next?

25

Existential Distress

The presentation of existential distress can be hard to identify, and for many people can oscillate between being very present and shifting away (usually in the context of medical things happening). Many people will recognize the presence of it but may not be able to clearly articulate or put language to the ways that this is showing up.

Peta is a 40-year-old woman with advanced disease. She has been attending therapy for some time in the years since her diagnosis, but she has continued to present with high levels of distress, particularly in the context of engaging with her medical care. Over the past months, she has been told that there are no further active treatment options, and she has been very hesitant to engage with the support of the palliative care service and is actively seeking out alternative therapy pathways since everyone has 'given up on her'. Her symptoms are poorly managed, and she is experiencing significant pain, insomnia and nausea, and looks increasingly unwell each time she presents to the clinic.

Peta: I just don't know why this has happened to me.
Therapist: What exactly?
Peta: Well, five years ago, when I was diagnosed, I was well
             and healthy. And now, look at me, everyone has given
             up on me, and it's all on me. Just like when I went to

DOI: 10.4324/9781003431640-30

that first doctor and they told me it was all in my head,
even though I had the bleeding. I just kept going back
to him over and over again, and he just kept dismissing
me. And what is going to happen now? I have to fix
this for myself, the doctors aren't doing anything.

Therapist: I notice that we are back in the story about how
things were before the diagnosis again? Did you
notice that has shown up again?

Peta: What do you mean?

Therapist: Do you recall that in our last session we spoke quite
a lot about the way that the situation has changed,
but something keeps pulling you back to the way
that things were before the diagnosis, even though
that was five years ago now?

Peta: Oh yeah, I do remember you saying that now that
you mention it. But, it's true, I just don't know why
this has happened to me? (Pauses and looks to
therapist)

Therapist: I don't have an answer to that Peta, but I also don't
want us to get caught up in this today. I think that if
there was an answer to be found, you would have
found it by now. (Pauses) I would instead like to
focus on why this thought keeps showing up?

Peta: Well, if I knew about why it had happened, then it
would all make sense.

Therapist: Okay, so let's imagine that I can give you an answer
to that question. What do you think might change
about the here and now? What do you think would
feel different?

Peta: Well, I would know what had caused it, and I would
have been able to change it. And then I wouldn't be
in this space.

Therapist: But, remember we can't go back in time, as much as
we would like to. And so I am more interested about
what would look different in the right here. The
disease would still be here, just you might have a bit
more of an idea about why, rather than it feeling like
it came from nowhere.

Peta: But I don't want to think about being here. Here is terrible.

Therapist: (Pauses) I see that Peta. But I also see how hard you are working to stay disconnected from it. And, that seems exhausting. Would you mind if I gave you some difficult words?

Peta: I guess not. (Looks away from the therapist)

Therapist: Sometimes it can feel hard to sit in this space, where we are flashing back to the past all the time. It makes me worried that we might run out of time to talk about the stuff that is coming up now.

Peta: What things, that I need to sort things out for myself.

Therapist: Do you think there is anything else?

Peta: (Pauses) You mean the death stuff.

Therapist: Maybe. How do you think it is showing up? The death stuff, I mean.

Peta: It's not. I won't let it.

Therapist: Why not?

Peta: (Sits silently for several moments before becoming teary) I don't want to.

Therapist: What would you think about the idea that this story about the past is showing up because your brain is working really hard not to go to the death stuff?

Peta: Does anyone want to go to that stuff?

Therapist: Some people. But mostly not. Most people want to run away from it, because it feels impossible to sit with it. But, the tricky thing is that if you are spending all of your time working hard to work against it, the thing itself doesn't change, if you could change your disease you would have, but it will do what it is going to do, but instead of being able to connect with the stuff that's important, you are fighting. And my bet is that that fight is exhausting.

Peta: But if I give in to it, then it will come for me. (Pauses for a long time) And I am not ready. I just want to go back to how it was before. Where I was well. I went to work, and I spent time arguing with my partner about stupid things. Now we don't argue at all, because you can't argue with a dying person, can you? Even when I am being horrible to him, I watch him biting his tongue. He says the same thing to me as you do, about not being caught in the past, and that I need to let it go.

Therapist: (Pauses) Do you think that there is anything that you could do that would make you feel ready?

Peta: No. I will fight against this until my last breath. But you think that's wrong, don't you? Do you think I should just give up?

Therapist: I think only you can know the answer to that – we never know what we will do until we are in a situation. But, I think there is a cost to being in this space – you are being pulled into this past space, and missing the now. I wonder whether that is what John is trying to communicate when he says that you are getting pulled into the past. I wonder if that is his way of saying, 'I see how hard this is, but I want to help you make sense of this'. I might be wrong about this, but as you speak it makes me wonder if the territory of what has happened is well traveled, but the territory of what is to come is feeling overwhelming and terrifying, so going back there feels safer? It gives you something to fight against. But the stuff that is to come – that is almost too big.

Case Study Reflections:

1. In Peta's case, what were the things that jumped out at you as you read through the case and the transcript?
2. What ACT-congruent frameworks/interventions do you notice in the discussion?
3. What, if any, different moves/directions would you have taken to the therapist?
4. How do you think the therapist feels about working with Peta?
5. Where do you think the role of relationship and self-compassion could/would show up between the therapist and Peta?

26

A Hard Decision

As we have discussed throughout the book, the conceptualisation and work with decision making with this group can be challenging. On the one hand, there is a necessity of acceptance of the choices they are faced with, where the situations that the person is faced with often leaves little option but to approach it with acceptance. Conversely for some, the idea of avoidance and wishful thinking will be loaded into the idea of projecting a future, and avoidance will appear to be a safer option for them emotionally.

Ben is living with metastatic disease, since his diagnosis six months ago. During this time, the team has identified that he has found it difficult to 'accept' what is going on but continually tells the team that he wants to stop treatment.

Ben: I just keep thinking that I want to stop. What's the point of continuing on when I know that it isn't fixing the disease? It is just making me miserable.

Therapist: Do you have a sense of what it would feel like to stop?

Ben: Not really. I think I would then just not have any hope at all. Even though I know that this isn't working, it does help my pain, but it isn't making the cancer any smaller. But maybe it is doing something you know, what would it look like if I stopped? Maybe the disease takes off, or maybe it doesn't.

DOI: 10.4324/9781003431640-31

Therapist: Does your doctor have a sense do you think? My guess is that it might be hard to predict ... .

Ben: (Laughs) If she does she isn't giving anything away. But, she isn't trying to talk me out of stopping, which makes me think that she doesn't think it is doing much.

Therapist: Would that change things, do you think? If she was really pushing you to do it?

Ben: (Pauses) I think it would mean that she thought it was worthwhile. I don't know whether she is giving it to me for the sake of it, while at the same time knowing it is futile. (Pauses) But then I guess the whole thing is futile, isn't it? The outcome is fixed.

Therapist: I am wondering if it might not be about the outcome – of course the outcome is a huge piece in this, and I don't want to disregard it, but I wonder whether it might be more helpful to think about the utility of the treatment.

Ben: What do you mean?

Therapist: Well, it seems like the treatment at the moment is giving you things – those things might not be about changing the outcome, but it is helping to manage your pain, and that means you get to spend time with the kids for that couple of weeks in between cycles before the pain returns. You have also mentioned before that those 'good weeks' feel okay, and you get to do the things that are on your list that we have talked about before. I guess my question would be, what would it mean to stop those things, rather than focusing on the treatment itself?

Ben: Well, they are going to stop anyway at some time.

Therapist: Sure. I guess thinking about it another way, does the cost of the treatment feel like a reasonable trade-off for the time that you get? Even if it is just for now?

Ben: The time that I have with the kids is always worth it but there are days where even that is so hard – and I find myself yelling at them. I don't want that to be the memories that they have of me, but I am so exhausted by the process.

Therapist: So, let's play it out. What would it look like for you if you did stop? Because you can, right now, you can tell your doctor you don't want anymore.

Ben: Then I would just die.

Therapist: And it's hard to know what that would look like. And my guess is that no one will be able to give you the specifics around that.

Ben: That feels overwhelming.

Therapist: How is the overwhelm showing up?

Ben: It's everywhere. In my body and in my brain. It's just a mess – it isn't thoughts or emotions, it's just too big.

Therapist: Mmmm.

Ben: I think it's worse – the idea that I would just opt out, even though it's hard.

Therapist: This might sound strange, but I wonder if the comfort is in the idea of opting out, rather than what it would actually look like to opt out.

Ben: Maybe. (Pauses) Both of them feel so difficult. It's hard to know.

Therapist: What would it look like to have a 100% conviction in either?

Ben: (Pauses) I don't know. Both of the options are loaded. The rock and the hard place – I know what that means now.

Therapist: I wonder if that's the bit that we can bring acceptance to – not the choice, but in recognising that neither choice will feel 100% right or comfortable – not because of you, but because of the nature of the thing itself.

Case Study Reflections:

1. In Ben's case, what do you think are the main things that he is grappling with?
2. What ACT congruent frameworks/interventions do you notice in the discussion?

3. What, if any, different moves/directions could you have taken this conversation?
4. How would you measure the success of the therapeutic work in this space?
5. How do you think the therapist feels in working with Ben?

27

When Death Takes Too Long

It is perhaps a strange idea, but one of the things that comes up in teams that work with people at the end of life is the very real recognition that sometimes the worst thing that happens to people isn't death – it is the suffering that precedes it. This is a complex idea, in which subjectivity becomes a significant factor – for instance, those who are in this space may find their own ideas about mortality and what a measure of a good life, and for that matter, a good death looks like. You may find that as a clinician you are challenged by the ways in which your patients present in this space, their level of acceptance (or otherwise) about the situations that they find themselves presented with, and the ways that they conceptualise their own process around dying.

Jane is a 36-year-old woman with incurable disease. She has been in hospital with intractable pain (that which is not responsive to pain relief strategies). Since coming onto the ward, she has had significant intervention including nerve blocks, anaesthetic and palliative care involvement as well as psychological support in attempting to support her in managing her pain. She is well connected with her therapist, and despite her pain (and the difficulty in engaging in therapy whilst in pain) she has continued to request review.

Jane: It's the pain again. I am feeling tortured. The only
          moments of respite I ever have is when I am knocked

DOI: 10.4324/9781003431640-32

out. (Crying out) Even now, I can't get a second's respite from this.

Therapist: I can see how hard it is for you each moment, even in the time since I have come in the room, I see the ways that it is making it almost impossible to focus on anything else, even for a second. I suspect that this might be a stupid question, but is anything helping at the moment?

Jane: (Moving uncomfortably) No. Well, I had a brief reprieve last night when the nurse put a hot pack on my neck, and for a couple of seconds it was almost too hot to stay there, and I could focus on that for a bit, and I was almost a bit hopeful that it would shift it, but then it was back, and it sounds stupid, but it was worse.

Therapist: That doesn't sound stupid at all. You allowed yourself to connect with a glimmer that things might be different.

Jane: I can't allow myself that kind of hope anymore. It was worse all last night – the pain, the thoughts all of it.

Therapist: When you say the thoughts, are we talking about the 'dark thoughts' that you had mentioned a couple of weeks ago? On those really bad days.

Jane: (Groans and shifts in bed) Kind of. This is going to sound really dark, but there isn't much time when I am not hoping that those bad thoughts happen now.

Therapist: The death stuff?

Jane: Yeah.

Therapist: It sounds like the fear of those thoughts has shifted?

Jane: It's another stupid thing (moving around in the bed). Do you mind passing that pillow across? (Positions pillow under her legs) Where was I?

Therapist: The ways that the thoughts have shifted?

Jane: Yeah. How long have I known you? Five years or so? Almost all of that time I have been fighting with you about not allowing these thoughts about death in – you have always wanted me to go there, and I have fought it. But now, they are there all the time. And it's not so bad.

Therapist: This might sound strange – but do they feel comforting?

Jane: You know what, they do. How is that? (Lets out a long scream of pain)

Therapist: Are you okay? Should we take a break?

Jane: No point. It isn't going to change. This is it, all day every day.

Therapist: I can see why the death thoughts might feel comforting right now.

Jane: Tell me about it. If I could end it right now, I would. But, I can't I am stuck here, until something breaks, or the tumours finally push into something that is going to kill me (yells out again). I wish for that every night when I go to sleep.

Therapist: What stops you ending it?

Jane: (Pauses) That's a good question. I could, couldn't I? I could ask the team for more drugs, and people have talked about being able to request terminal sedation – but how would I know when the right time is? I can make sense of just going off to sleep one day and not waking up, but actively deciding to do it ... I don't know. That feels like something else.

Therapist: It's the ultimate control decision, isn't it? I think most people would find it hard to make that call – but it sounds like you are sitting in a really tough space between having an option, but that option not being a good option either. It doesn't feel like there is an easy path. And you know what I always say about the algebra stuff ... .

Jane: (Moaning) I know, while the pain is punching me in the face, it's almost impossible to work through this.

Therapist: Yup. I don't think that anyone could make these decisions easily at any time, let alone in the face of what you are managing – and all of the stuff that comes with it. The pain is the rock in the pond – but it brings with it anxiety, sleep deprivation, desperation, panic, and a million other things.

Jane: You must be so sick of me talking about this.

Therapist: I absolutely am not (laughs), but I am curious as to why you might think that?

Jane: (Moaning and shouting out with a spasm) There isn't anything that you can do with this, just like everyone else. This is just my lot now.

Questions for reflection:

1. What comes up for you in reading through this transcript? Did you notice anything about your own ideas or beliefs coming up?
2. What ACT principals, or ACT-congruent ideas, did you identify? (This might be less obvious than in other cases we have talked about).
3. What would you have done? Where might you have taken a different path than the therapist?
4. What do you identify of the 'stuckness' either for the patient, or the therapist?
5. How might it feel to be in the room with someone like Jane?

Conclusion

In the writing of this guide, I was hoping for a couple of things. Firstly, the book would be able to walk with people through the practicalities of working therapeutically with people at the end of life – some of these considerations are about the physicality of what it means to be approaching death, but equally about how to apply the familiar therapeutic approaches we know and understand into a space that is changeable, complex and often unfixable.

Secondly, that in approaching this work, you as the reader will have also have the opportunity to reflect not only on the concrete aspects of your practice, but more importantly on the other bits – the difficult spaces, the unknowingness, our own messy ideas and experiences with death and mortality, and the grief that shows up in therapy. As I write this, I think about how easily the reflections on the hard stuff might show up – the sense of not doing enough, or perhaps not showing up the way that you would imagine. I suspect the reflections about the value of the work, or how you have shown up well in the hardest of spaces might be the much quieter of the voices.

ACT provides a helpful and appropriate framework in which to work with the things that arise from approaching the end of life. But it also provides a framework for us as therapists – often in parallel to the experiences that our patients are having when they enter the therapy room. I would encourage you to lean into this, rather than to pull away, whether that be as a therapist, or as a human. It is sometimes in these spaces of discomfort that the most rewarding therapeutic work is done.

As we have reached the end of the book, I would encourage you to consciously think about how you integrate such practice into your day-to-day work. It may be that you are working in an acute care setting where therapeutic work is

DOI: 10.4324/9781003431640-33

ad hoc and feels chaotic, or it may be in a clinic room with a long-term patient who is unexpectedly faced with their mortality, and a million places in between. Regardless, I hope that there has been something that you can take along with you on the journey.

References

Arch, J.J., Fishbein, J.N., Ferris, M.C., Mitchell, J.L., Levin, M.E., Slivjak, E.T., Andorsky, D.J. and Kutner, J.S., 2020. Acceptability, feasibility, and efficacy potential of a multimodal acceptance and commitment therapy intervention to address psychosocial and advance care planning needs among anxious and depressed adults with metastatic cancer. *Journal of palliative medicine*, *23*(10), pp.1380–1385.

Bai, Z., Luo, S., Zhang, L., Wu, S. and Chi, I., 2020. Acceptance and commitment therapy (ACT) to reduce depression: A systematic review and meta-analysis. *Journal of affective disorders*, *260*, pp.728–737.

Byock, I.R., 1996. The nature of suffering and the nature of opportunity at the end of life. *Clinics in geriatric medicine*, *12*(2), pp.237–252.

Coto-Lesmes, R., Fernández-Rodríguez, C. and González-Fernández, S., 2020. Acceptance and commitment therapy in group format for anxiety and depression. A systematic review. *Journal of affective disorders*, *263*, pp.107–120.

Dahl, J. and Lundgren, T., 2006. Acceptance and commitment therapy (ACT) in the treatment of chronic pain. *Mindfulness-based treatment approaches: Clinician's guide to evidence base and applications*, pp.285–306.

Davis, E.L., Deane, F.P. and Lyons, G.C., 2019. An acceptance and commitment therapy self-help intervention for carers of patients in palliative care: Protocol of a feasibility randomised controlled trial. *Journal of health psychology*, *24*(5), pp.685–704.

Davis, E.L., Deane, F.P., Lyons, G.C., Barclay, G.D., Bourne, J. and Connolly, V., 2020. Feasibility randomised controlled trial of a self-help acceptance and commitment therapy intervention for grief and psychological distress in carers of palliative care patients. *Journal of health psychology*, *25*(3), pp.322–339.

Davis, E.L., Deane, F.P., Lyons, G.C. and Barclay, G.D., 2017. Is higher acceptance associated with less anticipatory grief among patients in palliative care? *Journal of pain and symptom management*, *54*(1), pp.120–125.

Emerson, N.D., Tabuenca, K. and Bursch, B., 2022. End-of-life care in patients with cancer 16–24 years of age. *Current oncology reports*, *24*(2), pp.195–202.

Fashler, S.R., Weinrib, A.Z., Azam, M.A. and Katz, J., 2018. The use of acceptance and commitment therapy in oncology settings: A narrative review. *Psychological reports*, *121*(2), pp.229–252.

Fernández-Rodríguez, C., González-Fernández, S., Coto-Lesmes, R. and Pedrosa, I., 2021. Behavioral activation and acceptance and commitment therapy in the treatment of anxiety and depression in cancer survivors: A randomized clinical trial. *Behavior modification*, *45*(5), pp.822–859.

Fisher, S., Gillanders, D. and Ferreira, N., 2022. The experiences of palliative care professionals and their responses to work-related stress: A qualitative study. *British journal of health psychology*, *27*(2), pp.605–622.

Fitchett, G., Hisey Pierson, A.L., Hoffmeyer, C., Labuschagne, D., Lee, A., Levine, S., O'Mahony, S., Pugliese, K. and Waite, N., 2020. Development of the PC-7, a quantifiable assessment of spiritual concerns of patients receiving palliative care near the end of life. *Journal of palliative medicine*, *23*(2), pp.248–253.

Finucane, A.M., Hulbert-Williams, N.J., Swash, B., Spiller, J.A., Wright, B., Milton, L. and Gillanders, D., 2023. Feasibility of RESTORE: An online acceptance and commitment therapy intervention to improve palliative care staff wellbeing. *Palliative medicine*, *37*(2), pp.244–256.

Fulton, J.J., Newins, A.R., Porter, L.S. and Ramos, K., 2018. Psychotherapy targeting depression and anxiety for use in palliative care: A meta-analysis. *Journal of palliative medicine*, *21*(7), pp.1024–1037.

Gibson-Watt, T., Gillanders, D., Spiller, J. and Finucane, A., 2022. P-71 Acceptance and commitment therapy (ACT) for people with palliative care needs, their caregivers and staff involved in their care: A systematic scoping review. *BMJ supportive & palliative care*, *12*(Suppl 2), pp.A35–A35.

Gloster, A.T., Walder, N., Levin, M.E., Twohig, M.P. and Karekla, M., 2020. The empirical status of acceptance and commitment therapy: A review of meta-analyses. *Journal of contextual behavioral science*, *18*, pp.181–192.

González-Fernández, S. and Fernández-Rodríguez, C., 2019. Acceptance and commitment therapy in cancer: Review of applications and findings. *Behavioral medicine*, *45*(3), pp.255–269.

Graham, C.D., Gouick, J., Krahé, C. and Gillanders, D., 2016. A systematic review of the use of acceptance and commitment therapy (ACT) in chronic disease and long-term conditions. *Clinical psychology review*, *46*, pp.46–58.

Gramling, R., Straton, J., Ingersoll, L.T., Clarfeld, L.A., Hirsch, L., Gramling, C.J., Durieux, B.N., Rizzo, D.M., Eppstein, M.J. and Alexander, S.C., 2021. Epidemiology of fear, sadness, and anger expression in palliative care conversations. *Journal of pain and symptom management*, *61*(2), pp.246–253.

Gudat, H., Ohnsorge, K., Streeck, N. and Rehmann-Sutter, C., 2019. How palliative care patients' feelings of being a burden to others can motivate a wish to die. *Moral challenges in clinics and families. Bioethics*, *33*(4), pp.421–430.

Guthrie, D., 2023. How I learned to stop worrying and love the eco-apocalypse: An existential approach to accepting eco-anxiety. *Perspectives on psychological science*, *18*(1), pp.210–223.

Hajatpour, R. and Rashidi, H.H., 2021. The effectiveness of acceptance and commitment therapy on irrational beliefs and death attitude in the elderly. *Aging psychology*, *7*(1), pp.43–54.

Han, A., Yuen, H.K. and Jenkins, J., 2021. Acceptance and commitment therapy for family caregivers: A systematic review and meta-analysis. *Journal of health psychology*, *26*(1), pp.82–102.

Harris, R., 2021. *The happiness trap: How to stop struggling and start living*. Exisle Publishing.

Harris, R., 2022. *The happiness trap: How to stop struggling and start living* (2nd ed). Exisle Publishing.

Harris, R., 2013. *Getting unstuck in ACT: A clinician's guide to overcoming common obstacles in acceptance and commitment therapy*. New Harbinger Publications.

Harris, R., 2019. *ACT made simple: An easy-to-read primer on acceptance and commitment therapy* (2nd ed.). New Harbinger Publications.

Hayes, S.C. and Strosahl, K.D. eds., 2004. *A practical guide to acceptance and commitment therapy*. Springer Science & Business Media.

Henson, L.A., Maddocks, M., Evans, C., Davidson, M., Hicks, S. and Higginson, I.J., 2020. Palliative care and the management of common distressing symptoms in advanced cancer: Pain, breathlessness, nausea and vomiting, and fatigue. *Journal of clinical oncology*, 38(9), p.905.

Hill, R.C., Dempster, M., Donnelly, M. and McCorry, N.K., 2016. Improving the wellbeing of staff who work in palliative care settings: A systematic review of psychosocial interventions. *Palliative medicine*, 30(9), pp.825–833.

Hulbert-Williams, N.J., Hulbert-Williams, L., Patterson, P., Suleman, S. and Howells, L., 2021. Acceptance and commitment therapy (ACT)-enhanced communication skills: Development and evaluation of a novel training programme. *BMJ supportive & palliative care.*

Hulbert-Williams, N.J., Storey, L. and Wilson, K.G., 2015. Psychological interventions for patients with cancer: Psychological flexibility and the potential utility of acceptance and commitment therapy. *European journal of cancer care*, 24(1), pp.15–27.

Hulbert-Williams, N.J., Norwood, S.F., Gillanders, D., Finucane, A.M., Spiller, J., Strachan, J., Millington, S., Kreft, J. and Swash, B., 2021. Brief engagement and acceptance coaching for hospice settings (the BEACHeS study): Results from a Phase I study of acceptability and initial effectiveness in people with non-curative cancer. *BMC palliative care*, 20(1), pp.1–13.

Hulbert-Williams, N.J., Norwood, S., Gillanders, D., Finucane, A., Spiller, J., Strachan, J., Millington, S. and Swash, B., 2019. Brief Engagement and Acceptance Coaching for Community and Hospice Settings (the BEACHeS Study): Protocol for the development and pilot testing of an evidence-based psychological intervention to enhance wellbeing and aid transition into palliative care. *Pilot and feasibility studies*, 5, pp.1–9.

Jones, K., Methley, A., Boyle, G., Garcia, R. and Vseteckova, J., 2022. A systematic review of the effectiveness of acceptance and commitment therapy for managing grief experienced by bereaved spouses or partners of adults who had received palliative care. *Illness, crisis & loss*, 30(4), pp.596–613.

Kluger, B.M., Garvan, C.W. and Holloway, R.G., 2021. Joy, suffering, and the goals of medicine. *JAMA neurology*, 78(3), pp.265–266.

Kozlov, E., Phongtankuel, V., Prigerson, H., Adelman, R., Shalev, A., Czaja, S., Dignam, R., Baughn, R. and Reid, M.C., 2019. Prevalence, severity, and correlates of symptoms of anxiety and depression at the very end of life. *Journal of pain and symptom management, 58*(1), pp.80–85.

Li, H., Wong, C.L., Jin, X., Chen, J., Chong, Y.Y. and Bai, Y., 2021. Effects of acceptance and commitment therapy on health-related outcomes for patients with advanced cancer: A systematic review. *International journal of nursing studies, 115*, p.103876.

Martin, C.L. and Pakenham, K.I., 2022. The role of psychological flexibility in palliative care. *Journal of contextual behavioral science, 24*, pp.160–170.

Mathew, A., Doorenbos, A.Z., Jang, M.K. and Hershberger, P.E., 2021. Acceptance and commitment therapy in adult cancer survivors: A systematic review and conceptual model. *Journal of cancer survivorship, 15*, pp.427–451.

McFarland, D.C., Walsh, L., Napolitano, S., Morita, J. and Jaiswal, R., 2019. Suicide in patients with cancer: Identifying the risk factors. *Oncology (08909091), 33*(6), pp.221–226.

Mitchell, A.J., Chan, M., Bhatti, H., Halton, M., Grassi, L., Johansen, C. and Meader, N., 2011. Prevalence of depression, anxiety, and adjustment disorder in oncological, haematological, and palliative-care settings: A meta-analysis of 94 interview-based studies. *The Lancet oncology, 12*(2), pp.160–174.

Montaner, X., Tárrega, S., Pulgarin, M. and Moix, J., 2022. Effectiveness of acceptance and commitment therapy (ACT) in professional dementia caregivers burnout. *Clinical gerontologist, 45*(4), pp.915–926.

Mosher, C.E., Secinti, E., Hirsh, A.T., Hanna, N., Einhorn, L.H., Jalal, S.I., Durm, G., Champion, V.L. and Johns, S.A., 2019. Acceptance and commitment therapy for symptom interference in advanced lung cancer and caregiver distress: A pilot randomized trial. *Journal of pain and symptom management, 58*(4), pp.632–644.

Mosher, C.E., Secinti, E., Wu, W., Kashy, D.A., Kroenke, K., Bricker, J.B., Helft, P.R., Turk, A.A., Loehrer, P.J., Sehdev, A. and Al-Hader, A.A., 2022. Acceptance and commitment therapy for patient fatigue interference and caregiver burden in advanced gastrointestinal cancer: Results of a pilot randomized trial. *Palliative medicine*, *36*(7), pp.1104–1117.

Nafilyan, V., Morgan, J., Mais, D., Sleeman, K.E., Butt, A., Ward, I., Tucker, J., Appleby, L. and Glickman, M., 2023. Risk of suicide after diagnosis of severe physical health conditions: A retrospective cohort study of 47 million people. *The Lancet regional health-Europe*, *25*, p.100562.

Neff, K., 2011. *Self-compassion: The proven power of being kind to yourself*. Hachette UK.

Nzwalo, I., Aboim, M.A., Joaquim, N., Marreiros, A. and Nzwalo, H., 2020. Systematic review of the prevalence, predictors, and treatment of insomnia in palliative care. *American journal of hospice and palliative medicine*, *37*(11), pp.957–969.

Nunziante, F., Tanzi, S., Alquati, S., Autelitano, C., Bedeschi, E., Bertocchi, E., Dragani, M., Simonazzi, D., Turola, E., Braglia, L. and Masini, L., 2021. Providing dignity therapy to patients with advanced cancer: A feasibility study within the setting of a hospital palliative care unit. *BMC palliative care*, *20*, pp.1–12.

O'Hayer, C.V.F., O'Hayer, K.M. and Sama, A., 2018. Acceptance and commitment therapy with pancreatic cancer: An integrative model of palliative care—A case report. *Journal of pancreatic cancer*, *4*(1), pp.1–3.

Parpa, E., Tsilika, E., Galanos, A., Nikoloudi, M. and Mystakidou, K., 2019. Depression as mediator and or moderator on the relationship between hopelessness and patients' desire for hastened death. *Supportive care in cancer*, *27*, pp.4353–4358.

Petkus, A.J. and Wetherell, J.L., 2013. Acceptance and commitment therapy with older adults: Rationale and considerations. *Cognitive and behavioral practice*, *20*(1), pp.47–56.

Ringel, S., 2001. In the shadow of death: Relational paradigms in clinical supervision. *Clinical social work journal*, *29*(2), pp.171–179.

Robb, H., 2007. Values as leading principles in acceptance and commitment therapy. *International journal of behavioral consultation and therapy*, *3*(1), p.118.

Rodríguez-Prat, A., Balaguer, A., Crespo, I. and Monforte-Royo, C., 2019. Feeling like a burden to others and the wish to hasten death in patients with advanced illness: A systematic review. *Bioethics*, *33*(4), pp.411–420.

Safari Mousavi, S.S., Ghazanfari, F. and Mirderikvandi, F., 2019. Effectiveness of acceptance and commitment therapy on death anxiety in women with multiple sclerosis in Khorramabad. *Journal of clinical nursing and midwifery, 7*(4), pp.234–241.

Salamanca-Balen, N., Merluzzi, T.V. and Chen, M., 2021. The effectiveness of hope-fostering interventions in palliative care: A systematic review and meta-analysis. *Palliative medicine, 35*(4), pp.710–728.

Serfaty, M., Armstrong, M., Vickerstaff, V., Davis, S., Gola, A., McNamee, P., Omar, R.Z., King, M., Tookman, A., Jones, L. and Low, J.T., 2019. Acceptance and commitment therapy for adults with advanced cancer (CanACT): A feasibility randomised controlled trial. *Psycho-oncology, 28*(3), pp.488–496.

Secinti, E., Tometich, D.B., Johns, S.A. and Mosher, C.E., 2019. The relationship between acceptance of cancer and distress: A meta-analytic review. *Clinical psychology review, 71*, pp.27–38.

Soleimani, M.A., Bahrami, N., Allen, K.A. and Alimoradi, Z., 2020. Death anxiety in patients with cancer: A systematic review and meta-analysis. *European journal of oncology nursing, 48*, p.101803.

Swain, J., Hancock, K., Hainsworth, C. and Bowman, J., 2013. Acceptance and commitment therapy in the treatment of anxiety: A systematic review. *Clinical psychology review, 33*(8), pp.965–978.

Thompson, E.M., Destree, L., Albertella, L. and Fontenelle, L.F., 2021. Internet-based acceptance and commitment therapy: A transdiagnostic systematic review and meta-analysis for mental health outcomes. *Behavior therapy, 52*(2), pp.492–507.

Twohig, M.P. and Levin, M.E., 2017. Acceptance and commitment therapy as a treatment for anxiety and depression: A review. *Psychiatric clinics, 40*(4), pp.751–770.

Warth, M., Kessler, J., Koehler, F., Aguilar-Raab, C., Bardenheuer, H.J. and Ditzen, B., 2019. Brief psychosocial interventions improve quality of life of patients receiving palliative care: A systematic review and meta-analysis. *Palliative medicine, 33*(3), pp.332–345.

Yalom, I.D., 2008. Staring at the sun: Overcoming the terror of death. *The humanistic psychologist, 36*(3–4), pp.283–297.

Zambrano, S.C., Chur-Hansen, A. and Crawford, G.B., 2014. The experiences, coping mechanisms, and impact of death and dying on palliative medicine specialists. *Palliative & supportive care*, *12*(4), pp.309–316.

Zhao, C., Lai, L., Zhang, L., Cai, Z., Ren, Z., Shi, C., Luo, W. and Yan, Y., 2021. The effects of acceptance and commitment therapy on the psychological and physical outcomes among cancer patients: A meta-analysis with trial sequential analysis. *Journal of psychosomatic research*, *140*, p.110304.

Index

For Product Safety Concerns and Information please contact our EU
representative GPSR@taylorandfrancis.com Taylor & Francis Verlag GmbH,
Kaufingerstraße 24, 80331 München, Germany

Printed and bound by CPI Group (UK) Ltd, Croydon, CR0 4YY
08/06/2025
01897005-0007